Cyber Trafficking, Threat Behavior, and Malicious Activity Monitoring for Healthcare Organizations

Dinesh C. Dobhal
Graphic Era University (Deemed), India

Sachin Sharma
Graphic Era University (Deemed), India

Kamlesh C. Purohit
Graphic Era University (Deemed), India

Lata Nautiyal
University of Bristol, UK

Karan Singh
Jawaharlal Nehru University, India

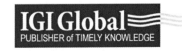

A volume in the Advances in Information Security, Privacy, and Ethics (AISPE) Book Series

Published in the United States of America by
  IGI Global
  Medical Information Science Reference (an imprint of IGI Global)
  701 E. Chocolate Avenue
  Hershey PA, USA 17033
  Tel: 717-533-8845
  Fax: 717-533-8661
  E-mail: cust@igi-global.com
  Web site: http://www.igi-global.com

Library of Congress Cataloging-in-Publication Data

Names: Dobhal, Dinesh C. (Dinesh Chandra), 1979- editor. I Sharma, Sachin,
   1988- editor. I Purohit, Kamlesh C. (Kamlesh Chandra), 1980- editor. I
   Nautiyal, Lata, 1980- editor. I Singh, Karan, 1981 May 20- editor.
Title: Cyber trafficking, threat behavior, and malicious activity
   monitoring for healthcare organizations / Dinesh C. Dobhal, Sachin
   Sharma, Kamlesh C. Purohit, Lata Nautiyal, and Karan Singh.
Description: Hershey PA : Medical Information Science Reference, [2023] I
   Includes bibliographical references and index. I Summary: "Cyber
   Trafficking, Threat Behavior, and Malicious Activity Monitoring for
   Healthcare Organizations provides a comprehensive review of techniques
   and applications of industry 5.0-enabled intelligent healthcare centric
   cyber security. The goal of this book is to close the gap between AI and
   cyber security. Covering topics such as malicious activity, dark web,
   and smart healthcare systems, this premier reference source is an
   essential resource for healthcare administrators, IT managers, system
   developers, system architects, IT specialists, students and educators of
   higher education, librarians, researchers, and academicians"-- Provided
   by publisher.
Identifiers: LCCN 2022046824 (print) I LCCN 2022046825 (ebook) I ISBN
   9781668466469 (hardcover) I ISBN 9781668466476 (ebook)
Subjects: MESH: Computer Security I Delivery of Health Care I Medical
   Informatics I Artificial Intelligence
Classification: LCC R859.7.A78 (print) I LCC R859.7.A78 (ebook) I NLM W
   26.55.C7 I DDC 362.10285--dc23/eng/20221209
LC record available at https://lccn.loc.gov/2022046824
LC ebook record available at https://lccn.loc.gov/2022046825

This book is published in the IGI Global book series Advances in Information Security, Privacy, and Ethics (AISPE) (ISSN: 1948-9730; eISSN: 1948-9749)

British Cataloguing in Publication Data
A Cataloguing in Publication record for this book is available from the British Library.

All work contributed to this book is new, previously-unpublished material.
The views expressed in this book are those of the authors, but not necessarily of the publisher.

For electronic access to this publication, please contact: eresources@igi-global.com.

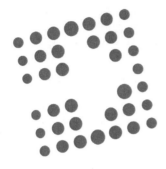

Advances in Information Security, Privacy, and Ethics (AISPE) Book Series

ISSN:1948-9730
EISSN:1948-9749

Editor-in-Chief: Manish Gupta, State University of New York, USA

MISSION

As digital technologies become more pervasive in everyday life and the Internet is utilized in ever increasing ways by both private and public entities, concern over digital threats becomes more prevalent.

The **Advances in Information Security, Privacy, & Ethics (AISPE) Book Series** provides cutting-edge research on the protection and misuse of information and technology across various industries and settings. Comprised of scholarly research on topics such as identity management, cryptography, system security, authentication, and data protection, this book series is ideal for reference by IT professionals, academicians, and upper-level students.

COVERAGE

- Electronic Mail Security
- Device Fingerprinting
- Internet Governance
- CIA Triad of Information Security
- Network Security Services
- Risk Management
- Computer ethics
- Privacy Issues of Social Networking
- Data Storage of Minors
- Security Classifications

IGI Global is currently accepting manuscripts for publication within this series. To submit a proposal for a volume in this series, please contact our Acquisition Editors at Acquisitions@igi-global.com or visit: http://www.igi-global.com/publish/.

Titles in this Series

For a list of additional titles in this series, please visit:
ttp://www.igi-global.com/book-series/advances-information-security-privacy-ethics/37157

Emerging Perspectives in Systems Security Engineering, Data Science, and Artificial Intelligence
Maurice Dawson (Illinois Institute of Technology, USA)
Information Science Reference • copyright 2023 • 315pp • H/C (ISBN: 9781668463253) • US $250.00 (our price)

Global Perspectives on the Applications of Computer Vision in Cybersecurity
Franklin Tchakounte (University of Ngaoundere, Cameroon) and Marcellin Atemkeng (University of Rhodes, South Africa)
Engineering Science Reference • copyright 2023 • 300pp • H/C (ISBN: 9781668481271) • US $250.00 (our price)

Handbook of Research on Data Science and Cybersecurity Innovations in Industry 4.0 Technologies
Thangavel Murugan (United Arab Emirates University, Al Ain, UAE) and Nirmala E. (VIT Bhopal University, India)
Information Science Reference • copyright 2023 • 600pp • H/C (ISBN: 9781668481455) • US $325.00 (our price)

Perspectives on Ethical Hacking and Penetration Testing
Keshav Kaushik (University of Petroleum and Energy Studies, India) and Akashdeep Bhardwaj (University of Petroleum and Energy Studies, India)
Information Science Reference • copyright 2023 • 300pp • H/C (ISBN: 9781668482186) • US $225.00 (our price)

Malware Analysis and Intrusion Detection in Cyber-Physical Systems
S. L. Shiva Darshan (Department of Information and Communication Technology, Manipal Institute of Technology, India) M. V. Manoj Kumar (Department of Information Science and Engineering, Nitte Meenakshi Institute of Technology, India) B. S. Prashanth (Department of

For an entire list of titles in this series, please visit:
ttp://www.igi-global.com/book-series/advances-information-security-privacy-ethics/37157

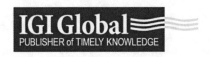

701 East Chocolate Avenue, Hershey, PA 17033, USA
Tel: 717-533-8845 x100 • Fax: 717-533-8661
E-Mail: cust@igi-global.com • www.igi-global.com

Table of Contents

Preface...xiii

Chapter 1
Advances of Cyber Security in the Healthcare Domain for Analyzing Data 1
    Guru Prasad M. S., Graphic Era University (Deemed), India
    Praveen Gujjar, Faculty of Management Studies, Jain University
        (Deemed), India
    H. N. Naveen Kumar, Vidyavardhaka College of Engineering, India
    M. Anand Kumar, School of Information Science, Presidency University,
        India
    S. Chandrappa, Jain University (Deemed), India

Chapter 2
Machine Learning-Based Cyber Intrusion Detection System for Internet of
Medical Things Attacks in Healthcare Environments 15
    Bhawnesh Kumar, Graphic Era University (Deemed), India
    Ashwani Kumar, Shri Ram Group of Colleges, India
    Harendra Singh Negi, Graphic Era University (Deemed), India
    Javed Alam, Quantlase Lab, Abu Dhabi, UAE

Chapter 3
Blockchain-Enabled Smart Healthcare Systems Using IoT.................................30
    Abhishek Kumar, School of Computer and Systems Sciences, Jawaharlal
        Nehru University, India
    Karan Singh, School of Computer and Systems Sciences, Jawaharlal
        Nehru University, India

Chapter 4
Significance of Cyber Security in Healthcare Systems.......................................51
    Anuj Singh, Graphic Era University (Deemed), India
    Somjit Mandal, National Chiao Tung University, Hsinchu, Taiwan
    Kamlesh Chandra Purohit, Graphic Era University (Deemed), India

Chapter 5
Secure Data Sharing Using Revocable-Storage Identity-Based Encryption........72
    Muthumanikandan Vanamoorthy, Vellore Institute of Technology,
       Chennai, India

Chapter 6
A Machine Learning-Based Framework for Intrusion Detection Systems in
Healthcare Systems 85
    Janmejay Pant, Graphic Era Hill University, India
    Rakesh Kumar Sharma, Pal College of Technology and Management,
       Haldwani, India
    Himanshu Pant, Graphic Era Hill University, India
    Devendra Singh, Graphic Era Hill University, India
    Durgesh Pant, Uttarakhand Open University, Haldwani, India

Chapter 7
Dispute Between Countries, a Corresponding Attack on Cyberspace: The
New National Security Challenge..96
    Siddhardha Kollabathini, Jawaharlal Nehru University, India

Chapter 8
A Review on Application of Reinforcement Learning in Healthcare................105
    Chitra A. Dhawale, P.R. Pote College of Engineering and Management,
       India
    Kritika Anil Dhawale, University of Technology Sydney, Australia

Chapter 9
Artificial Intelligence: A Tool for Detection of Pandemics 120
    Kumud Pant, Graphic Era University (Deemed), India
    Bhasker Pant, Graphic Era University (Deemed), India
    Somya Sinha, Graphic Era University (Deemed), India

Chapter 10
Cyberstalking: Consequences and Coping Strategies to Improve Mental
Health...143
    Abhishek Bansal, Indira Gandhi National Tribal University,
       Amarkantak, India
    Arvind Kumar Gautam, Indira Gandhi Naitonal Tribal University,
       Amarkantak, India
    Sudesh Kumar, Indira Gandhi Naitonal Tribal University, Amarkantak,
       India

Compilation of References 172

About the Contributors 203

Index 205

Detailed Table of Contents

Preface xiii

Chapter 1

Advances of Cyber Security in the Healthcare Domain for Analyzing Data 1

Guru Prasad M. S., Graphic Era University (Deemed), India
Praveen Gujjar, Faculty of Management Studies, Jain University
(Deemed), India
H. N. Naveen Kumar, Vidyavardhaka College of Engineering, India
M. Anand Kumar, School of Information Science, Presidency University,
India
S. Chandrappa, Jain University (Deemed), India

Analyzing healthcare data is an important part of improving patient outcomes and driving healthcare innovation. With the increasing digitization of healthcare records and the growing use of electronic health records (EHRs), there is a wealth of data available that can be used to inform clinical decision-making. Analyzing healthcare data comes with its own unique set of challenges. Healthcare data can be complex and voluminous, and it often exists in disparate systems and formats. Cybersecurity is becoming increasingly important in the healthcare domain, as the industry is rapidly digitizing and relying more on electronic data management systems. This chapter analyzed the current state of cybersecurity in the healthcare domain, discussing the common types of cyber threats faced by healthcare organizations and the potential impact of these threats on patient care. The goal of this chapter is to provide an overview of healthcare data analysis and to highlight the ways in which security feature can be used to drive improvements in patient care and healthcare outcomes.

Chapter 2

Machine Learning-Based Cyber Intrusion Detection System for Internet of
Medical Things Attacks in Healthcare Environments 15

Bhawnesh Kumar, Graphic Era University (Deemed), India
Ashwani Kumar, Shri Ram Group of Colleges, India
Harendra Singh Negi, Graphic Era University (Deemed), India
Javed Alam, Quantlase Lab, Abu Dhabi, UAE

In this chapter, the authors calculate the accuracy value of machine learning models for combined, network, bio-medical data. The result shows that random forest has the highest accuracy value 94.17% for combined and 93.19% bio-medical data. For network data, decision tree classifier provides the highest accuracy value which is 94.07% whereas decision tree regression gives the highest accuracy value: 94.62% for combined, 92.11% for bio-medical, and 94.09% for network data.

Chapter 3
Blockchain-Enabled Smart Healthcare Systems Using IoT.................................30
Abhishek Kumar, School of Computer and Systems Sciences, Jawaharlal Nehru University, India
Karan Singh, School of Computer and Systems Sciences, Jawaharlal Nehru University, India

A healthcare system is the medical platform through which patients get better treatment. Several hospitals and doctors are linked together through this platform in a hierarchy and treat the patient easily. In view of the COVID-19 pandemic, it is a very challenging task to treat the patients physically; therefore, there is a need to redevelop the healthcare system to fulfill the modern demand. The state of the art of this scheme is to provide remote treatment facilities and build a secure online system. Blockchain technology combined with IoT provides the solution through its vital features of transparency, immutability, decentralization, and trust-less environment. IoT devices capture the patient health status and process it and send to blockchain; therefore, information sharing between devices, hospitals, and doctors are at risk and need to provide security. Using key management scheme in smart contract to ensure integrity of data, this scheme provides better treatment at cheap cost as well as efficiency and security compared to traditional healthcare systems.

Chapter 4
Significance of Cyber Security in Healthcare Systems..51
Anuj Singh, Graphic Era University (Deemed), India
Somjit Mandal, National Chiao Tung University, Hsinchu, Taiwan
Kamlesh Chandra Purohit, Graphic Era University (Deemed), India

The healthcare sector is one of the industries most vulnerable to cyberattacks. healthcare cybercrime is significantly expanding as it relates to healthcare services that are digitally enabled, and it aims to exploit security flaws and vulnerabilities. Technology improvements have exposed the healthcare sector to a wide range of extremely dangerous threats, such as ransomware. Ransomware, a sort of hack that targets both organisations and individual people, has become more prevalent recently as a result of its effective results. There has been a significant improvement in its disputes over the previous several years. The study includes answers as well as a complete overview of ransomware attacks. The main goal of this study is to classify the cyberattack defences employed by healthcare programmes to stop ransomware, such as blockchain and machine learning. Studies investigating information security, medical organisations, and security firms will all benefit scientifically from the study.

Chapter 5

Secure Data Sharing Using Revocable-Storage Identity-Based Encryption........72
Muthumanikandan Vanamoorthy, Vellore Institute of Technology, Chennai, India

Distributed computing provides flexible and informative information exchange and brings many benefits to both the general public and individuals. However, because the information often contains the most important data, there is a common lock that allows users to easily reuse cloud host information. Therefore, it is important for users to provide cryptographically enhanced access control to shared resources. Personality-based encryption is, for example, a promising encryption approach for building smart data sharing systems. Anyway, access to management is not a versatile solution. In such cases, if your permission is revoked from the database, it must be completely revoked from the cloud server, and you will not be able to retrieve your information once it has been revoked. It has many features of realizability, usefulness, and effectiveness and thus shows the correlation that shows the proposed method diagram used to build a practical and intelligent data provider structure.

Chapter 6

A Machine Learning-Based Framework for Intrusion Detection Systems in Healthcare Systems...85
Janmejay Pant, Graphic Era Hill University, India
Rakesh Kumar Sharma, Pal College of Technology and Management, Haldwani, India
Himanshu Pant, Graphic Era Hill University, India
Devendra Singh, Graphic Era Hill University, India
Durgesh Pant, Uttarakhand Open University, Haldwani, India

A reliable intrusion detection system is an important key component of healthcare-based systems. Intrusion detection systems are crucial in e-healthcare because patient medical records must be maintained accurately, safely, and secretly. Errors in diagnosis and therapy might result from changing the actual patient data. It is not possible to handle complex data using traditional techniques. Current network requirements cannot be met by diversified intrusion techniques. In addition to the rise in data, attacks are also escalating rapidly. The area of network security is trending when it comes to machine learning techniques. This study aims to develop a novel machine learning framework for detecting attacks.

Chapter 7

Dispute Between Countries, a Corresponding Attack on Cyberspace: The
New National Security Challenge 96
Siddhardha Kollabathini, Jawaharlal Nehru University, India

Today, cyberspace is a fact of daily life, and cyberspace's impact has not bypassed
states' national security. Cyberspace, a manmade technological advancement over
the past decades, transformed the way economies work around the world, reshaping
social interactions and a paradigm shift in politics. Cyberspace being boundaryless,
omnipresent across multiple domains, and anarchic has been considered to attack
whenever there are any disputes between two countries. In the context described
above, a pressing question arises. Cyberspace is not a domain like land, water and
air, and it is an environment inhabited by information and knowledge, existing in
electronic form. If cyberspace is a mere inhabitation of information and knowledge,
why do states want to consider cyberspace as an arena for confrontation in any dispute
between countries? This chapter proposes discussing this new phenomenon, looking
into the evaluation and analysing aspects of the recent phenomenon.

Chapter 8

A Review on Application of Reinforcement Learning in Healthcare 105
*Chitra A. Dhawale, P.R. Pote College of Engineering and Management,
        India*
Kritika Anil Dhawale, University of Technology Sydney, Australia

We are witnessing the era of data science where data is generating in an exponential
manner. This big data is working as fuel to explore the business in every domain
and healthcare is not the exception for this. Data analysis and data analytics in
collaboration with machine learning techniques are playing an important role in
every domain. Supervised and unsupervised approaches in machine learning depends
on one shot, exhaustive, and reward output. Reinforcement learning (RL) handles
these issues with sequential decision making problems, concurrent evaluation, and
feedback methods. RL technique can be a suitable candidate for developing powerful
solutions in a variety of healthcare domains. This chapter will focus on the broad
applications of RL techniques in healthcare domains, which can be helpful to the
researchers with systematic understanding of conceptual information, techniques,
and an overview of RL applications in healthcare domains for various types of
diseases right from chronic diseases and mental disorder.

Chapter 9

Artificial Intelligence: A Tool for Detection of Pandemics 120
Kumud Pant, Graphic Era University (Deemed), India
Bhasker Pant, Graphic Era University (Deemed), India
Somya Sinha, Graphic Era University (Deemed), India

The spread of the COVID-19 pandemic made us rethink the need for integrating modern scientific algorithms in decision support as well as medical systems. This chapter focuses on the on-going efforts throughout the world for tackling the COVID-19 pandemic with the use of artificial intelligence and machine learning algorithms. The chapter also compiles the various efforts made internationally for providing solution to this disease. The examples of use of algorithms like artificial neural network, fuzzy clustering, and support vector machines for both the disease recognition as well as in medical aid have been stated. Finally, the chapter also reiterates the need for developing even more advanced algorithms and prediction systems in case of future pandemic outbreaks due to ever mutating microorganisms and other lifestyle problems. More than just scientific and governmental endeavors, prudent handling of any emergency health situation requires awareness as well as self-discipline exercised by inhabitants of any country.

Chapter 10
Cyberstalking: Consequences and Coping Strategies to Improve Mental Health 143
> *Abhishek Bansal, Indira Gandhi National Tribal University, Amarkantak, India*
> *Arvind Kumar Gautam, Indira Gandhi Naitonal Tribal University, Amarkantak, India*
> *Sudesh Kumar, Indira Gandhi Naitonal Tribal University, Amarkantak, India*

Cyberstalking is one of the most widespread threats on digital platforms. It has included many forms of direct threats via email, online distribution of intimate photographs, seeking information about victims, harassment, and catfishing. The consequences of cyberstalking may lead to psychological problems such as mental health, distress, victim experiencing feelings of isolation, guilt, adverse effects on life activity. These psychological problems may further lead to reports of serious health issues such as anger, fear, suicidal ideation, depression, and post-traumatic stress disorder (PTSD). However, there are many coping strategies such as avoidant coping, ignoring the perpetrator, confrontational coping, support seeking, and cognitive reframing. In spite of these methods, awareness of preventive measures of cyberstalking may further help to overcome mental stress. In this chapter, the authors have pointed out the various psychological issues due to cyberstalking and further discuss their solutions through preventing or automatic detection methods inspired by machine learning approaches.

Compilation of References 172

About the Contributors 203

Index 205

Preface

In today's rapidly evolving digital landscape, research plays a crucial role in addressing the pressing challenges faced by healthcare organizations in the realm of cyber security. As the healthcare sector embraces the advancements of Industry 5.0, the need for innovative solutions that leverage artificial intelligence becomes paramount. This edited reference book, titled "Cyber Trafficking, Threat Behavior, and Malicious Activity Monitoring for Healthcare Organizations," serves as a valuable resource that not only highlights the importance of research but also provides practical insights and techniques to tackle these challenges head-on.

The significance of research in the context of cyber security and healthcare cannot be overstated. Traditional security solutions have proven insufficient in the face of the ever-evolving cyber threat landscape. With cybercrime becoming more sophisticated, it is imperative to explore new methodologies and technologies that can effectively combat these threats. The chapters presented in this book aim to bridge the gap between artificial intelligence and cyber security, demonstrating how innovative research can contribute to the protection of healthcare organizations and their valuable data.

By addressing a wide range of topics, this book offers a comprehensive review of the techniques and applications of Industry 5.0 enabled Intelligent Healthcare centric Cyber Security. Each chapter presents cutting-edge research developments, highlighting the potential applications of artificial intelligence, machine learning, blockchain technology, and data-driven network intelligence, among others. Through these advancements, readers are empowered to develop innovative solutions that can effectively detect and prevent cyber trafficking, threat behavior, and malicious activities within healthcare organizations.

Furthermore, this book not only serves as a valuable resource for academic courses in Information Systems and Technologies, Business Process Management, and Cybersecurity, but also as a guide for senior executives, IT professionals, and researchers. It provides them with the necessary tools and knowledge to understand the intricacies of cyber security in the healthcare sector and to navigate the challenges posed by Industry 5.0.

We firmly believe that research is the key to solving the outlined problems in cyber security for healthcare organizations. The insights and methodologies presented in this book will empower the readers to develop robust and intelligent systems that can effectively protect healthcare data, identify vulnerabilities, detect fraud, and ensure the integrity of healthcare networks. By encouraging further research, innovation, and collaboration, this book aims to propel the field of Industry 5.0 enabled Intelligent Healthcare centric Cyber Security forward, fostering a safer and more secure environment for healthcare organizations and their stakeholders.

We extend our gratitude to the contributing authors whose expertise and dedication have made this book possible. Their valuable insights and research contributions are instrumental in advancing the field of cyber security in healthcare.

We hope that this edited reference book will serve as a catalyst for further research, inspire new ideas, and drive the development of innovative solutions that address the complex challenges faced by healthcare organizations in the ever-evolving digital landscape.

CHAPTER OVERVIEW

Chapter 1: Advances of Cyber Security in Healthcare Domain for Analyzing the Data

In this chapter, authored by Guru Prasad M S, Praveen Gujjar, Naveen Kumar, Anand Kumar M, and Chadnrappa S, the focus is on the crucial role of cybersecurity in the healthcare domain and its impact on data analysis. The authors acknowledge the increasing digitization of healthcare records and the growing reliance on electronic health records (EHRs) to inform clinical decision-making. However, they highlight the unique challenges associated with analyzing healthcare data, such as its complexity, volume, and the existence of disparate systems and formats.

The chapter delves into the current state of cybersecurity in the healthcare domain, shedding light on the common types of cyber threats faced by healthcare organizations. It emphasizes the potential impact of these threats on patient care, thereby underlining the critical need for robust cybersecurity measures. The authors aim to provide an overview of healthcare data analysis, illustrating how security features can be effectively utilized to drive improvements in patient care and overall healthcare outcomes.

By exploring the intersection of cybersecurity and data analysis in the healthcare domain, this chapter serves as an important foundation for understanding the significance of protecting healthcare data while leveraging it for meaningful insights. The insights presented in this chapter will inform readers about the current state of cybersecurity in healthcare and provide valuable guidance on utilizing security features to enhance patient care and healthcare outcomes.

Chapter 2: Machine Learning-Based Cyber Intrusion Detection System for Internet of Medical Things Attacks in Healthcare Environments

Authored by Bhawnesh Kumar, Ashwani Kumar, Harendra Singh Negi, and Javed Alam, this chapter focuses on the development of a machine learning-based cyber intrusion detection system (IDS) specifically designed to mitigate attacks on the Internet of Medical Things (IoMT) in healthcare environments.

The authors acknowledge the increasing adoption of sensor-based devices in advanced healthcare systems, which enable the collection of patient details from remote locations through the internet. These IoMT devices play a crucial role in facilitating the collection of patient data, which can then be utilized for making predictions and informed decisions in the future treatment plans of patients. However, the transmission and storage of patient data via the internet pose significant security risks that need to be addressed.

The chapter proposes the integration of machine learning models into existing healthcare systems, along with an intrusion detection system, to enhance the security and quality of healthcare services. The authors evaluate the accuracy of machine learning models using combined, network, and bio-medical data. The results demonstrate that the random forest model achieves the highest accuracy value of 94.17% for combined data and 93.19% for bio-medical data. Additionally, the decision tree classifier exhibits the highest accuracy value of 94.07% for network data, while the decision tree regression model achieves the highest accuracy value of 94.62% for combined data, 92.11% for bio-medical data, and 94.09% for network data.

By developing and evaluating machine learning-based models for cyber intrusion detection in IoMT environments, this chapter provides valuable insights into enhancing the security and integrity of healthcare systems. The presented results highlight the potential of machine learning techniques, such as random forest and decision tree algorithms, to effectively detect and mitigate attacks on the IoMT infrastructure in healthcare environments. This chapter serves as a resource for researchers and practitioners interested in developing robust intrusion detection systems for securing medical IoT devices and safeguarding patient data in healthcare settings.

Chapter 3: Blockchain-Enabled Smart Healthcare System Using IoT

Authored by Abhishek Kumar and Karan Singh, this chapter focuses on the development of a blockchain-enabled smart healthcare system that leverages the Internet of Things (IoT) to address the challenges faced by the healthcare industry. The authors recognize the importance of a robust healthcare system that can efficiently connect hospitals, doctors, and patients, especially in the context of the COVID-19 pandemic.

The chapter emphasizes the need to redevelop the healthcare system to meet modern demands, including the provision of remote treatment facilities and the establishment of a secure online platform. To achieve these goals, the authors propose combining blockchain technology with IoT. Blockchain technology offers essential features such as transparency, immutability, decentralization, and a trustless environment, which can significantly enhance the security and efficiency of the healthcare system.

In the proposed scheme, IoT devices capture and process the health status of patients, transmitting the data to the blockchain. This ensures secure information sharing between devices, hospitals, and doctors, mitigating the risks associated with data privacy and security. The authors highlight the importance of utilizing key management schemes in smart contracts to ensure the integrity of the data stored on the blockchain.

By implementing a blockchain-enabled smart healthcare system using IoT, this chapter presents a solution that provides improved treatment facilities at a lower cost compared to traditional healthcare systems. The integration of blockchain and IoT technologies enables enhanced security, efficiency, and transparency in the healthcare ecosystem. This chapter serves as a valuable resource for researchers and practitioners interested in exploring the potential of blockchain and IoT in revolutionizing healthcare systems and delivering more accessible and secure healthcare services.

Chapter 4: Significance of Cyber Security in Healthcare Systems

Authored by Anuj Singh, Somjit Mandal, and Kamlesh Chandra Purohit, this chapter sheds light on the critical significance of cyber security in the healthcare system. The authors highlight the healthcare sector's vulnerability to cyberattacks, emphasizing the expanding nature of healthcare cybercrime and its exploitation of security flaws and vulnerabilities.

With advancements in technology, the healthcare sector has become increasingly exposed to a wide range of highly dangerous threats, particularly ransomware. Ransomware attacks, which target both organizations and individuals, have gained prominence due to their effectiveness in recent years. The chapter provides a comprehensive overview of ransomware attacks, offering insights into their nature, trends, and evolving characteristics.

The primary objective of this study is to classify the cyberattack defenses employed by healthcare programs to prevent ransomware attacks. The authors explore the potential of technologies such as blockchain and machine learning in enhancing cyber security measures within the healthcare system. By investigating information security, medical organizations, and security firms, the study contributes scientifically to the understanding and improvement of cyber security in the healthcare domain.

This chapter serves as a valuable resource for researchers and professionals in the field of healthcare cyber security. By highlighting the significance of cyber security in healthcare systems and examining defense mechanisms against ransomware attacks, this chapter aims to raise awareness about the importance of robust security measures and the potential of advanced technologies in safeguarding sensitive healthcare data. The insights presented in this chapter will contribute to the scientific understanding of cyber security in healthcare and assist in the development of effective strategies to combat cyber threats in the industry.

Chapter 5: Secure Data Sharing Using Revocable-Storage Identity-Based Encryption

Authored by Muthumanikandan Vanamoorhty, this chapter focuses on the secure sharing of data through the utilization of revocable-storage identity-based encryption. The author acknowledges the benefits of distributed computing in facilitating flexible and informative information exchange for both the public and individuals. However, the sensitivity of the shared data often necessitates robust access control measures to prevent unauthorized reuse or access by cloud hosts.

Identity-based encryption, specifically revocable-storage identity-based encryption, is proposed as a promising cryptographic approach for building intelligent data sharing systems. The chapter highlights the importance of providing users with cryptographically enhanced access control to shared resources. While access management is a versatile solution, there are cases where revocation of permissions is necessary. In such instances, if a user's permission is revoked from the database, it should be completely revoked from the cloud server, ensuring that the user can no longer retrieve the information once it has been revoked.

The proposed method described in this chapter demonstrates the feasibility, utility, and effectiveness of the revocable-storage identity-based encryption approach. It presents a practical and intelligent data provider structure that addresses the need for secure data sharing. By utilizing revocable-storage identity-based encryption, the chapter offers insights into constructing a system that enhances the security and control of shared data.

This chapter serves as a valuable resource for researchers and practitioners interested in secure data sharing and access control mechanisms. The proposed revocable-storage identity-based encryption approach presented in this chapter contributes to the development of practical and intelligent data sharing systems, ensuring secure and controlled data access while allowing for efficient revocation when necessary. The insights provided in this chapter will help advance the field of secure data sharing and contribute to the development of robust cryptographic solutions in distributed computing environments.

Chapter 6: A Machine Learning-Based Framework for Intrusion Detection Systems in Healthcare Systems

Authored by Janmejay Pant, Rakesh Kumar Sharma, Himanshu Pant, Devendra Singh, and Durgesh Pant, this chapter focuses on the development of a machine learning-based framework for intrusion detection systems in healthcare systems. The authors emphasize the importance of reliable intrusion detection systems as key components of healthcare-based systems, particularly in ensuring the accuracy, safety, and confidentiality of patient medical records.

Traditional techniques often struggle to handle the complexity of healthcare data, and the existing intrusion detection techniques fail to meet the evolving network requirements and the increasing number of attacks. In this context, the utilization of machine learning techniques has gained significant attention in the field of network security.

The chapter aims to develop a novel machine learning framework that effectively detects and mitigates attacks in healthcare systems. By leveraging machine learning algorithms, the framework offers the potential for improved accuracy and efficiency in intrusion detection. It addresses the challenges of complex healthcare data and the growing number of attacks by incorporating machine learning techniques into the intrusion detection process.

By developing this machine learning-based framework, the authors contribute to the advancement of intrusion detection systems in healthcare. The framework has the potential to enhance the security and integrity of healthcare systems, ensuring the reliability and confidentiality of patient data.

This chapter serves as a valuable resource for researchers and practitioners interested in the application of machine learning techniques in intrusion detection systems for healthcare environments. The proposed framework provides a foundation for developing more robust and efficient systems to combat the evolving threats faced by healthcare systems. The insights and methodologies presented in this chapter will contribute to the improvement of intrusion detection in healthcare settings, ultimately leading to more secure and reliable healthcare systems.

Chapter 7: Dispute Between Countries, a Corresponding Attack on Cyberspace – The New National Security Challenge

Authored by Siddhardha Kollabathini, this chapter explores the complex relationship between disputes between countries and corresponding attacks on cyberspace, presenting a new national security challenge. The chapter recognizes the omnipresence and transformative impact of cyberspace in our daily lives, as well as its influence on national security considerations.

Cyberspace, as a man-made technological advancement, has reshaped economies, social interactions, and politics worldwide. However, its boundaryless and anarchic nature has made it susceptible to attacks whenever disputes arise between countries. This raises an important question: If cyberspace is primarily an environment inhabited by information and knowledge in electronic form, why do states view it as an arena for confrontation during disputes?

The chapter aims to explore this new phenomenon by examining the evaluation and analysis of aspects related to the intersection of disputes between countries and attacks on cyberspace. By delving into the complexities and motivations behind this trend, the chapter sheds light on the evolving nature of national security challenges in the digital age.

This chapter serves as a thought-provoking resource for researchers and policymakers interested in understanding the implications of cyber conflicts in the context of international disputes. By examining this phenomenon, the chapter contributes to a deeper understanding of the dynamics between cyberspace and national security, encouraging further analysis and exploration of this evolving challenge.

Chapter 8: A Review on the Application of Reinforcement Learning in Healthcare

Authored by Chitra A. Dhawale and Kritika Anil Dhawale, this chapter provides a comprehensive review of the application of reinforcement learning (RL) techniques in the healthcare domain. The authors highlight the exponential growth of data in the era of data science and emphasize its significance in exploring business opportunities across various domains, including healthcare.

Data analysis, data analytics, and machine learning techniques have become integral components in leveraging the potential of big data. While supervised and unsupervised approaches in machine learning rely on one-shot, exhaustive outputs, and reward mechanisms, RL techniques address the challenges associated with sequential decision-making problems, concurrent evaluation, and feedback methods.

The chapter discusses how RL can serve as a suitable approach for developing powerful solutions in various healthcare domains. It explores the broad applications of RL techniques, providing researchers with a systematic understanding of the conceptual information, techniques, and an overview of RL applications in healthcare. The applications range from addressing chronic diseases to mental disorders, offering potential solutions for a wide range of healthcare challenges.

By reviewing and analyzing the application of RL in healthcare, this chapter contributes to the advancement of research in this field. It provides valuable insights into the potential of RL techniques to enhance healthcare outcomes and addresses various types of diseases. Researchers and practitioners in healthcare and machine learning will benefit from the comprehensive understanding and overview of RL applications in healthcare domains presented in this chapter.

Chapter 9: Artificial Intelligence: A Tool for Detection of Pandemic

Authored by Kumud Pant, Bhasker Pant, and Somya Sinha, this chapter explores the integration of modern scientific algorithms, specifically artificial intelligence (AI) and machine learning, in addressing the COVID-19 pandemic. The authors highlight the ongoing global efforts to combat the pandemic through the use of AI and machine learning algorithms.

The chapter compiles various international initiatives and solutions aimed at tackling the disease. It showcases the application of algorithms such as artificial neural networks, fuzzy clustering, and support vector machines in disease recognition and medical aid. These algorithms play a significant role in analyzing large amounts of data, identifying patterns, and providing decision support in the fight against the pandemic.

Additionally, the chapter emphasizes the need for the development of more advanced algorithms and prediction systems to prepare for future pandemic outbreaks. The ever-mutating nature of microorganisms and other lifestyle problems necessitates continuous advancements in AI and machine learning to effectively address and respond to such emergencies.

The authors underscore that, beyond scientific and governmental endeavors, handling emergency health situations like a pandemic requires awareness and self-discipline from the inhabitants of any country. This collective effort is crucial in implementing preventive measures and following guidelines to minimize the spread of the disease.

By highlighting the role of AI and machine learning in pandemic detection and management, this chapter contributes to the understanding of the potential of these technologies in public health emergencies. It emphasizes the importance of continued research and development to strengthen our ability to combat future pandemics effectively. The insights presented in this chapter will be valuable to researchers, policymakers, and healthcare professionals involved in utilizing AI tools for pandemic detection and response.

Chapter 10: Cyberstalking – Consequences and Coping Strategies to Improve Mental Health

Authored by Abhishek Bansal, Arvind Kumar Gautam, and Sudesh Kumar, this chapter addresses the widespread threat of cyberstalking on digital platforms and its detrimental consequences. Cyberstalking encompasses various forms of direct threats, including email harassment, the online distribution of intimate photographs, seeking personal information about victims, and engaging in harassment and catfishing.

The consequences of cyberstalking extend beyond digital platforms and can have profound psychological effects on the victims. These effects include mental health issues, distress, feelings of isolation, guilt, and adverse impacts on daily life activities. In severe cases, cyberstalking can lead to serious health issues such as anger, fear, suicidal ideation, depression, and post-traumatic stress disorder (PTSD).

To address these psychological challenges, coping strategies are essential. This chapter explores various coping strategies, including avoidant coping, ignoring the perpetrator, confrontational coping, support seeking, and cognitive reframing.

These strategies can help victims mitigate the impact of cyberstalking and improve their mental well-being.

Additionally, the chapter emphasizes the importance of awareness and preventive measures to combat cyberstalking and reduce mental stress. It discusses the potential of machine learning approaches for automatic detection methods, which can contribute to early intervention and prevention of cyberstalking incidents.

By shedding light on the psychological issues arising from cyberstalking and discussing coping strategies and preventive measures, this chapter provides valuable insights into the impact of cyberstalking on mental health and ways to mitigate its effects. The information presented will be beneficial for researchers, practitioners, and individuals seeking to understand and address the challenges posed by cyberstalking, ultimately promoting improved mental health and well-being in the digital age.

IN SUMMARY

In conclusion, this edited reference book delves into the critical intersection of cyber security and healthcare, providing a comprehensive overview of the challenges, advancements, and applications in this domain. The chapters presented in this book offer valuable insights into various aspects of cyber security in healthcare, ranging from data analysis and intrusion detection to the integration of artificial intelligence and machine learning techniques.

Throughout the book, we have explored the significance of research in addressing the outlined problems and finding innovative solutions. The chapters highlight the importance of leveraging modern technologies, such as blockchain, IoT, reinforcement learning, and artificial intelligence, to enhance cyber security measures and improve patient care outcomes.

The contributions from the authors have covered a wide range of topics, including the analysis of healthcare data, machine learning-based intrusion detection systems, blockchain-enabled smart healthcare systems, and the role of artificial intelligence in pandemic detection. Each chapter offers unique perspectives, methodologies, and practical applications that contribute to the body of knowledge in this field.

We believe that this edited reference book will serve as a valuable resource for researchers, practitioners, and professionals in the fields of healthcare, cyber security, information systems, and technology. The comprehensive review of techniques, frameworks, and development tools, along with the exploration of cutting-edge research developments, will empower readers to innovate in cyber security applications within the healthcare sector.

We extend our gratitude to all the authors who have contributed their expertise and insights to this book. Their dedication and contributions have enriched the content and ensured the provision of valuable information to our readers.

It is our hope that this book will inspire further research, collaboration, and advancements in the field of cyber security in healthcare. As technology continues to evolve, so too must our strategies and solutions to safeguard sensitive healthcare data and protect patient well-being.

We encourage readers to delve into the chapters and explore the diverse perspectives presented in this book. By leveraging the knowledge and insights shared within these pages, we can collectively work towards a future where cyber security in healthcare is robust, resilient, and capable of ensuring the highest standards of patient care and data protection.

Thank you for joining us on this journey of exploring cyber security, threat behavior monitoring, and malicious activity detection for healthcare organizations.

Dinesh C. Dobhal
Graphic Era University (Deemed), India

Sachin Sharma
Graphic Era University (Deemed), India

Kamlesh C. Purohit
Graphic Era University (Deemed), India

Lata Nautiyal
University of Bristol, UK

Karan Singh
Jawaharlal Nehru University, India

Chapter 1
Advances of Cyber Security in the Healthcare Domain for Analyzing Data

Guru Prasad M. S.
iD https://orcid.org/0000-0002-1811-9507
Graphic Era University (Deemed), India

Praveen Gujjar
Faculty of Management Studies, Jain University (Deemed), India

H. N. Naveen Kumar
Vidyavardhaka College of Engineering, India

M. Anand Kumar
School of Information Science, Presidency University, India

S. Chandrappa
Jain University (Deemed), India

ABSTRACT

Analyzing healthcare data is an important part of improving patient outcomes and driving healthcare innovation. With the increasing digitization of healthcare records and the growing use of electronic health records (EHRs), there is a wealth of data available that can be used to inform clinical decision-making. Analyzing healthcare data comes with its own unique set of challenges. Healthcare data can be complex and voluminous, and it often exists in disparate systems and formats. Cybersecurity is becoming increasingly important in the healthcare domain, as the industry is rapidly digitizing and relying more on electronic data management systems. This chapter analyzed the current state of cybersecurity in the healthcare domain, discussing the common types of cyber threats faced by healthcare organizations and the potential

DOI: 10.4018/978-1-6684-6646-9.ch001

impact of these threats on patient care. The goal of this chapter is to provide an overview of healthcare data analysis and to highlight the ways in which security feature can be used to drive improvements in patient care and healthcare outcomes.

INTRODUCTION

The healthcare industry is increasingly relying on digital technologies to manage and analyze patient data, which has led to an exponential increase in the volume and complexity of healthcare data. However, this digitization also poses a significant threat to the confidentiality, integrity, and availability of healthcare data, making the healthcare sector one of the most targeted industries for cyber-attacks. Cybersecurity breaches in healthcare can have dire consequences, including identity theft, financial fraud, loss of trust, and even harm to patients. Therefore, healthcare organizations must adopt robust cybersecurity measures to protect sensitive data from cyber threats. This includes implementing best practices such as strong access controls, encryption, regular vulnerability assessments, and employee training programs. In addition to these preventative measures, data analysis can also play a critical role in healthcare cybersecurity. By analyzing healthcare data, organizations can identify potential vulnerabilities, detect anomalous behavior, and respond to incidents quickly and effectively. Data analysis techniques such as machine learning and artificial intelligence can help organizations identify patterns and trends in data that may be indicative of cyber-attacks. Healthcare organizations must also consider the ethical implications of data analysis, particularly when it comes to protecting patient privacy. Data anonymization and de-identification techniques must be used to ensure that sensitive patient data is not compromised during the analysis process. Healthcare organizations must take a proactive approach to cybersecurity, implementing strong protective measures and leveraging data analysis to detect and respond to threats. With the increasing reliance on technology in healthcare, cybersecurity must be a top priority to ensure the confidentiality, integrity, and availability of healthcare data and the safety and wellbeing of patients.

CYBERSECURITY AND HEALTH CARE DOMAIN

The healthcare industry is increasingly digitized, with healthcare organizations relying on electronic health records (EHRs), telemedicine, and other digital technologies to manage patient data and provide care. While these technologies bring many benefits, they also create new cybersecurity risks. Healthcare data is highly valuable on the black market, making healthcare organizations a prime target for cyber criminals (J. Agarwal, 2023). Cybersecurity breaches in healthcare can have serious consequences, including compromised patient data, financial losses, and reputational damage. Additionally, cyber-attacks can impact patient care, leading to disruptions in service and even harm to patients. Therefore, healthcare organizations must prioritize cybersecurity to protect sensitive data and ensure the safety and wellbeing of patients. Some of the specific cybersecurity risks facing healthcare organizations include ransomware attacks, phishing, and insider threats. Cyber criminals may use these tactics to gain access to healthcare data, disrupt healthcare services, or even extort organizations for ransom payments. Healthcare organizations must implement strong protective measures, such as firewalls, intrusion detection systems, and data encryption, to prevent these types of attacks. In addition to these preventative measures, healthcare organizations can also leverage data analysis to detect and respond to cyber threats. By analyzing healthcare data, organizations can identify patterns and trends that may be indicative of an attack and respond quickly and effectively. Healthcare organizations must also prioritize employee training and awareness programs to ensure that all staff members are aware of cybersecurity risks and how to protect sensitive data. This includes educating staff members on how to identify and respond to phishing attacks and other cybersecurity threats. Cybersecurity is an essential aspect of healthcare in the digital age. Healthcare organizations must take proactive measures to protect sensitive data and ensure the safety and wellbeing of patients. This includes implementing strong protective measures, leveraging data analysis, and prioritizing employee training and awareness programs.

RELATED WORKS

More than ever, medical organizations need to priorities cybersecurity. The high risk for cybersecurity places are primary healthcare consultancies, diagnostic service provider, academic, and research enterprises, etc. (Tully et al., 2020; Coronado & Wong, 2014). By installing security measures that use strong authentication mechanisms in conjunction with staff training, a crucial follow-up activity that some firms prefer to ignore at the risk of becoming a headline in cybersecurity, the possibility of a breach is reduced. Cybercriminals commonly take advantage of a particular weakness in the healthcare industry to weaken the company's supply chain. Health organizations maintain a wide network in which enormous volumes of data are continually exchanged since they depend on several external services and providers (Coronado & Wong, 2014; Strielkina et al., 2018; Kruse et al., 2017). As the healthcare sector grows more technologically connected, cybercrime risk rises. The two categories of stealing are internal and external. Hackers that are not connected to the healthcare sector infiltrate patient and medical systems in order to steal and acquire data, mainly for financial benefit. They could make false insurance claims using the patient's confidential information. Hackers may demand a ransom from healthcare organizations in order to restore patient data systems as an additional form of external theft. A whole system could be compromised by sophisticated malware and phishing techniques that collect login information or install malicious applications on a computer. The fact that malware can infiltrate a network with just one seemingly trustworthy link is one of the trickiest aspects of dealing with it (Argaw et al., 2020; Choi & Johnson, 2021). One of the main reasons for the high death rate in the globe is cancer. By recognizing the cancer disease in its earliest stages, this can be reduced. Since the lungs are one of the most common cancer locations, lung cancer is taken into account in the proposed study. The lungs' X-ray images are employed in the proposed study to find the malignant tumour in its earliest stages. X-ray pictures of the chest are segmented using Otsu's thresholding technique. The components of the feature vector are the numbers of white and black pixels and the histogram characteristics of the segmented image. Utilizing feature vectors, the Feed-Forward Neural Network with Back Propagation (FFNN-BP) and K-Nearest Neighbourhood Classifier (KNNC) classify tumours as benign or malignant (Avinash et al., 2023). Attacks can be happened for the AI and ML models which is called as adversarial attacks. The trained model can also be vulnerable for theses adversarial attacks (Gujjar, J. P 2021). The chatbot can be used to respond for security concern of the user. (Gujjar, P., & HR, P. K. (2022, December). The users related queries can easily have resolved with the help of specific chatbot (Jagannath, P. G.et al 2022).

CHARACTERISTICS OF CYBERSECURITY IN HEALTH CARE DOMAIN

Cybersecurity in the healthcare domain is a complex and dynamic field that presents several unique characteristics and challenges. Some of the key characteristics of cybersecurity in healthcare include:

1. Sensitive data: Healthcare data is some of the most sensitive and confidential information, including health information and personal information. This makes healthcare organizations a prime target for cybercriminals who seek to obtain this data for financial gain or other nefarious purposes.
2. Complexity: The healthcare industry is highly complex, with multiple stakeholders and systems involved in delivering care and managing patient

data. This complexity makes it challenging to implement and maintain effective cybersecurity measures, particularly in legacy systems.

3. Limited resources: Healthcare organizations often have limited resources to devote to cybersecurity, particularly in smaller practices or hospitals. This can make it difficult to implement and maintain robust cybersecurity measures.

4. Insider threats: Insider threats, such as employee negligence or malicious activity, are a significant concern in healthcare cybersecurity. Healthcare organizations must implement strong access controls and employee training programs to mitigate these threats.

5. Connected devices: The Internet of Things (IoT) has led to an increasing number of connected medical devices, which can present cybersecurity risks. These devices may not have strong security measures in place, making them vulnerable to cyber-attacks.

Cybersecurity in the healthcare domain is a multifaceted and constantly evolving field. Healthcare organizations must address these unique characteristics and challenges to effectively protect sensitive data and ensure the safety and wellbeing of patients.

ADVANCES OF CYBERSECURITY IN ANALYZING THE DATA

Advances in cybersecurity have enabled healthcare organizations to analyze healthcare data more effectively while maintaining the privacy and security of patient information. Some of the key advances in cybersecurity that have enabled more secure and effective data analysis in healthcare include:

1. Encryption: Encryption is a crucial cybersecurity tool that can help protect sensitive data while it is being transmitted or stored. Advances in encryption technology have made it possible to encrypt data at rest and in transit, making it more difficult for cybercriminals to access and steal healthcare data.

2. Anonymization and de-identification: Anonymization and de-identification techniques allow healthcare organizations to analyze healthcare data without compromising patient privacy. These techniques remove or obscure identifiable information from data sets, allowing for safe and ethical analysis.

3. Machine learning: Machine learning is a powerful tool for analyzing large amounts of healthcare data quickly and efficiently. Advances in machine learning algorithms have made it possible to detect patterns and trends in data that may be indicative of cyber-attacks or other security threats.

4.   Artificial intelligence (AI): AI can help healthcare organizations detect and respond to cyber threats more quickly and effectively. AI algorithms can analyze data in real-time, identify anomalies and suspicious behavior, and alert security teams to potential threats.

5.   Cloud computing: Cloud computing can provide healthcare organizations with a more secure and scalable way to store and analyze healthcare data. Cloud providers typically offer robust security measures, such as data encryption and access controls, to protect sensitive data.

ADVANTAGES OF CYBERSECURITY IN HEALTHCARE DOMAIN FOR ANALYZING THE DATA

Cybersecurity in the healthcare domain plays a critical role in protecting patient data and ensuring the safety and wellbeing of patients. In addition, cybersecurity also provides several advantages for analyzing healthcare data. Some of the key advantages of cybersecurity in healthcare domain for analyzing data include: Protecting sensitive data: Cybersecurity measures protect sensitive healthcare data from cyber-attacks and breaches (P. M. S. Guru, 2023). By implementing strong security measures, healthcare organizations can ensure that patient data is kept confidential and secure, which is essential for ethical and legal reasons. Ensuring data integrity: Cybersecurity measures can help to ensure the integrity of healthcare data. Data integrity ensures that healthcare data is accurate, consistent, and reliable, making it easier to analyze and derive meaningful insights. Enabling data sharing: Cybersecurity measures can facilitate the secure sharing of healthcare data between healthcare organizations, researchers, and other stakeholders. This enables more collaborative and effective data analysis, which can lead to better patient outcomes. Improving patient outcomes: By analyzing healthcare data, healthcare organizations can identify patterns and trends that can help improve patient outcomes. This includes identifying new treatments and therapies, predicting disease outbreaks, and optimizing healthcare delivery. Supporting regulatory compliance: Healthcare organizations are subject to numerous regulations and standards related to data privacy and security, including HIPAA, HITECH, and GDPR. Cybersecurity measures can help healthcare organizations comply with these regulations, avoiding costly penalties and reputational damage. Cybersecurity in healthcare domain provides significant advantages for analyzing healthcare data. By protecting sensitive data, ensuring data integrity, enabling data sharing, improving patient outcomes, and supporting regulatory compliance, cybersecurity plays a crucial role in advancing healthcare research and delivery.

ADVANCES OF HEALTHCARE DOMAIN FOR ANALYZING THE DATA

The healthcare domain has made significant advances in analyzing healthcare data in recent years, which has enabled healthcare organizations to derive valuable insights from healthcare data to improve patient care and outcomes (M. A. Kumar, 2023). Some of the key advances in healthcare domain for analyzing data include: Electronic Health Records (EHRs): Electronic Health Records have replaced paper-based systems, providing a more efficient way to store and manage patient data. EHRs enable healthcare providers to access and analyze patient data more easily, leading to more accurate and timely diagnoses and treatments. Big Data Analytics: Big Data Analytics is a powerful tool for analyzing large amounts of healthcare data quickly and efficiently. By identifying patterns and trends in healthcare data, healthcare providers can develop more effective treatments and therapies, predict disease outbreaks, and optimize healthcare delivery. Real-time Data Analysis: Real-time data analysis allows healthcare providers to analyze patient data in real-time, enabling faster diagnosis and treatment decisions. This can be particularly important in emergency situations where every minute counts. Wearable Devices and Remote Monitoring: Wearable devices and remote monitoring technologies enable healthcare providers to collect real-time data on patients outside of traditional healthcare settings. This data can be used to identify trends and patterns, enabling more personalized and effective healthcare delivery. Precision Medicine: Precision medicine is a personalized approach to healthcare that is based on an individual's genetic makeup and other unique characteristics. By analyzing healthcare data at a molecular level, healthcare providers can develop more personalized and effective treatments.

NEED FOR CYBERSECURITY IN HEALTHCARE

Medical institutions can now treat patients, access shared data, and communicate with patients and staff using connected devices thanks to technological breakthroughs. All of the aforementioned skills, meanwhile, carry some danger. That risk is significantly reduced by a dependable, knowledgeable partner who understands compliance. The healthcare industry is of special interest to malicious hackers. Because fraudsters constantly search for vulnerabilities in healthcare systems, cybersecurity in healthcare is crucial for contact information, personal data, social security numbers, and banking information [10]. Cybersccurity is crucial in the healthcare industry due to the sensitivity and personal nature of healthcare data. Healthcare data typically includes personal and confidential information such as medical records, test results, and payment information, which makes it a prime target for cybercriminals. The need for cybersecurity in healthcare is driven by several factors, including: Protecting patient privacy: Healthcare data contains highly sensitive information that needs to be protected to maintain patient privacy. Cybersecurity measures are necessary to prevent unauthorized access, theft, or misuse of this information. Avoiding data breaches: Cyber-attacks can result in significant data breaches that can have serious consequences for patients and healthcare organizations. Cybersecurity measures can help to prevent data breaches, which can be costly both financially and in terms of reputational damage. Ensuring patient safety: Healthcare cybersecurity is essential to ensure patient safety. Cyber-attacks can disrupt healthcare services, compromise medical devices, and interfere with patient care, putting patients at risk. Compliance with regulations: Healthcare organizations are subject to numerous regulations related to data privacy and security, such as HIPAA and GDPR (M. S. Guru Prasad, 2023). Compliance with these regulations is necessary to avoid legal penalties and reputational damage. Protecting intellectual property: Healthcare organizations also need to protect their intellectual property, including research data and proprietary technologies. Cybersecurity measures can help to prevent intellectual property theft and protect against industrial espionage. The need for cybersecurity in healthcare is critical to protect patient privacy, avoid data breaches, ensure patient safety, comply with regulations, and protect intellectual property. Cybersecurity measures are essential for maintaining trust in the healthcare industry and ensuring that patients receive safe and effective care. The cybersecurity in healthcare domain involves antitheft device, disaster recovery plan, digital forensics, threat intelligence, vulnerability scans, data loss prevention etc., as shown in Figure 1.

ROLES OF CYBERSECURITY IN HEALTHCARE DOMAIN

The role of cybersecurity in the healthcare domain is critical in protecting sensitive patient data, maintaining patient privacy, ensuring patient safety, and protecting healthcare organizations from cyber threats. The cyber security roles are shown in Figure 2.

Figure 1. Cybersecurity smart tools

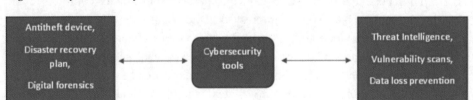

Figure 2. Cybersecurity roles in healthcare domain

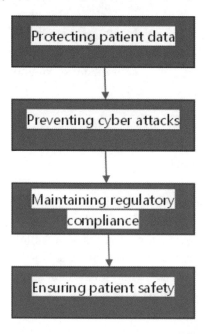

A. Protecting patient data: Cybersecurity plays a crucial role in protecting patient data from theft, unauthorized access, and misuse. Healthcare organizations must implement robust cybersecurity measures to secure patient data, including data encryption, firewalls, and intrusion detection and prevention systems.

B. Preventing cyber-attacks: Cybersecurity is essential for preventing cyber-attacks that can result in data breaches, network downtime, and other serious consequences. Healthcare organizations must implement security controls such as access controls, patch management, and security awareness training to reduce the risk of cyber-attacks (M. Anand Kumar, 2022).

C. Maintaining regulatory compliance: Healthcare organizations are subject to numerous regulations related to data privacy and security, such as HIPAA and GDPR. Compliance with these regulations is necessary to avoid legal penalties and reputational damage. Cybersecurity plays a crucial role in maintaining regulatory compliance by implementing security controls and conducting regular security audits.

D. Ensuring patient safety: Cybersecurity is essential for ensuring patient safety by protecting medical devices from cyber threats. Medical devices are increasingly connected to the internet, creating new vulnerabilities that can be exploited by cybercriminals. Cybersecurity measures can help to protect medical devices from cyber-attacks and prevent disruption to patient care.

CYBERSECURITY THREATS IN HEALTHCARE DOMAIN

The healthcare domain is particularly vulnerable to cybersecurity threats due to the highly sensitive nature of healthcare data and the increasing use of digital technology in healthcare (Singh. P, 2023). Some of the most common cybersecurity threats in the healthcare domain shown in Table 1.

FUTURE SCOPE FOR CYBERSECURITY IN HEALTHCARE DOMAIN

The future scope for cybersecurity in the healthcare domain is vast and will continue to grow as the healthcare industry increasingly relies on digital technology and data-driven insights. Here are some potential areas of future growth for cybersecurity in healthcare: Artificial Intelligence (AI) and Machine Learning (ML): AI and ML can be used to detect and prevent cyber threats in healthcare networks by analyzing patterns and identifying potential risks (A. P. H, 2023). As the use of AI and ML in healthcare continues to grow, cybersecurity tools that leverage these technologies will become more prevalent. Blockchain technology: Blockchain technology has the potential to improve the security and privacy of healthcare data by providing

Table 1. Cybersecurity threat

Sl.No	Cybersecurity Threat	Description
1	Ransomware attacks	Ransomware attacks are a significant threat to healthcare organizations, where cybercriminals encrypt data and demand payment in exchange for decryption. Ransomware attacks can disrupt healthcare services, compromise patient data, and result in significant financial losses.
2	Phishing attacks	Phishing attacks are commonly used by cybercriminals to gain access to healthcare networks. These attacks involve sending emails or messages that appear to be from a legitimate source, such as a healthcare organization or government agency. Once the recipient clicks on a malicious link or downloads an attachment, the attacker gains access to the network.
3	Insider threats	Insider threats are a significant risk in healthcare, where employees or contractors may intentionally or unintentionally compromise patient data. Insider threats can be caused by human error, negligence, or malicious intent.
4	Malware attacks	Malware attacks are a common threat in healthcare, where cybercriminals use malicious software to gain access to healthcare networks and data. Malware can be used to steal patient data, disrupt healthcare services, or compromise medical devices.
5	Internet of Things (IoT) attacks	IoT attacks are a growing concern in healthcare, where medical devices and other IoT devices are connected to healthcare networks. IoT devices are often vulnerable to cyber-attacks due to inadequate security controls, making them an easy target for cybercriminals.

a tamper-proof and transparent record of transactions. Blockchain-based solutions can help to prevent data breaches and protect patient privacy. Cloud-based security solutions: As healthcare organizations continue to move their data and applications to the cloud, cloud-based security solutions will become increasingly important. Cloud-based security solutions can provide scalable and flexible security controls that can adapt to changing threats and business needs. Advanced authentication methods: Advanced authentication methods, such as biometric authentication and multi-factor authentication, can improve the security of healthcare data by adding an extra layer of protection against unauthorized access (Prasad. G, 2019). Cybersecurity workforce development: With the increasing demand for cybersecurity professionals in healthcare, there will be a growing need for cybersecurity workforce development programs. These programs can help to train and educate cybersecurity professionals on the unique challenges and requirements of healthcare cybersecurity (N. H. R, 2022). The future scope for cybersecurity in healthcare is vast and will continue to grow as the healthcare industry evolves. As healthcare organizations continue to adopt digital technologies and data-driven insights, cybersecurity will become increasingly important for protecting patient data, maintaining regulatory compliance, and ensuring patient safety.

CONCLUSION

Businesses in the healthcare industry are particularly susceptible to cyberattacks because they hold a plethora of data that has significant financial and intelligence value to cybercriminals and nation-state actors. The goals of the pharmaceutical and healthcare industries are to save lives. It's a noble endeavor. They also deal with increasingly computerized personal and sensitive data. The advances of cybersecurity in the healthcare domain for analyzing data have significant benefits for healthcare organizations, patients, and the healthcare industry as a whole. With the increasing use of digital technology in healthcare, robust cybersecurity measures are essential for protecting patient data, maintaining regulatory compliance, and ensuring patient safety. The benefits of cybersecurity in healthcare include improved data protection, reduced risk of cyber-attacks, increased patient trust, and better patient outcomes. As the healthcare industry continues to evolve, the future scope for cybersecurity in healthcare is vast, with the potential for AI and ML, blockchain technology, cloud-based security solutions, advanced authentication methods, and cybersecurity workforce development programs. It is imperative for healthcare organizations to prioritize cybersecurity measures to ensure that patient data is secure and confidential, and the healthcare industry continues to provide quality care to patients.

REFERENCES

Abraham, C., Chatterjee, D., & Sims, R. R. (2019). Muddling through cybersecurity: Insights from the US healthcare industry. *Business Horizons*, *62*(4), 539–548. doi:10.1016/j.bushor.2019.03.010

Agarwal, J., Christa, S. A., Pai, H., & Kumar. (2023). Machine Learning Application for News Text Classification. *13th International Conference on Cloud Computing, Data Science & Engineering (Confluence)*, 463-466. 10.1109/Confluence56041.2023.10048856

Anand Kumar, M., Abirami, N., Guru Prasad, M. S., & Mohankumar, M. (2022). Stroke Disease Prediction based on ECG Signals using Deep Learning Techniques. *2022 International Conference on Computational Intelligence and Sustainable Engineering Solutions (CISES)*, 453-458. 10.1109/CISES54857.2022.9844403

Anandkumar, Agarwal, & Christa. (2023). Designing a Secure Audio / Text Based Captcha Using Neural Network. *2023 13th International Conference on Cloud Computing, Data Science & Engineering (Confluence)*, 510-514. 10.1109/Confluence56041.2023.10048791

Argaw, S. T., Troncoso-Pastoriza, J. R., Lacey, D., Florin, M. V., Calcavecchia, F., Anderson, D., & Flahault, A. (2020). Cybersecurity of Hospitals: Discussing the challenges and working towards mitigating the risks. *BMC Medical Informatics and Decision Making*, *20*(1), 1–10. doi:10.118612911-020-01161-7 PMID:32620167

Avinash, S., Naveen Kumar, H. N., Guru Prasad, M. S., Mohan Naik, R., & Parveen, G. (2023). Early Detection of Malignant Tumor in Lungs Using Feed-Forward Neural Network and K-Nearest Neighbor Classifier. *SN Computer Science*, *4*(2), 195. doi:10.100742979-022-01606-y

Burrell, D. N., Aridi, A. S., McLester, Q., Shufutinsky, A., Nobles, C., Dawson, M., & Muller, S. R. (2021). Exploring System Thinking Leadership Approaches to the Healthcare Cybersecurity Environment. *International Journal of Extreme Automation and Connectivity in Healthcare*, *3*(2), 20–32. doi:10.4018/IJEACH.2021070103

Choi, S. J., & Johnson, M. E. (2021). The relationship between cybersecurity ratings and the risk of hospital data breaches. *Journal of the American Medical Informatics Association : JAMIA*, *28*(10), 2085–2092. doi:10.1093/jamia/ocab142 PMID:34338786

Coronado, A. J., & Wong, T. L. (2014). Healthcare cybersecurity risk management: Keys to an effective plan. *Biomedical Instrumentation & Technology*, *48*(s1), 26–30. doi:10.2345/0899-8205-48.s1.26 PMID:24848146

Guru, P. M. S., Praveen, G. J., Dodmane, R., Sardar, T. H., Ashwitha, A., & Yeole, A. N. (2023). Brain Tumor Identification and Classification using a Novel Extraction Method based on Adapted Alexnet Architecture. *6th International Conference on Information Systems and Computer Networks (ISCON),* 1-5. 10.1109/ISCON57294.2023.10112075

Guru, P. M. S., Praveen, G. J., Dodmane, R., Sardar, T. H., Ashwitha, A., & Yeole, A. N. (2023). Brain Tumor Identification and Classification using a Novel Extraction Method based on Adapted Alexnet Architecture. *6th International Conference on Information Systems and Computer Networks (ISCON),* 1-5. 10.1109/ISCON57294.2023.10112075

Guru Prasad, M. S., Agarwal, J., Christa, S., Aditya Pai, H., Kumar, M. A., & Kukreti, A. (2023). An Improved Water Body Segmentation from Satellite Images using MSAA-Net. *2023 International Conference on Machine Intelligence for GeoAnalytics and Remote Sensing (MIGARS),* 1-4. 10.1109/MIGARS57353.2023.10064508

Guru Prasad, M. S., Naveen Kumar, H. N., Raju, K., Santhosh Kumar, D. K., & Chandrappa, S. (2023). Glaucoma Detection Using Clustering and Segmentation of the Optic Disc Region from Retinal Fundus Images. *SN Computer Science, 4*(2), 192. doi:10.100742979-022-01592-1

Kirubasri, G., Sankar, S., & Guru Prasad, M. S. (2023). *LQETA-RP: link quality based energy and trust aware routing protocol for wireless multimedia sensor networks.* Int J Syst Assur Eng Manag. doi:10.100713198-023-01873-9

Kruse, C. S., Frederick, B., Jacobson, T., & Monticone, D. K. (2017). Cybersecurity in healthcare: A systematic review of modern threats and trends. *Technology and Health Care, 25*(1), 1–10. doi:10.3233/THC-161263 PMID:27689562

Kumar, M. A., Pai, A. H., Agarwal, J., Christa, S., Prasad, G. M. S., & Saifi, S. (2023). *Deep Learning Model to Defend against Covert Channel Attacks in the SDN Networks. In Advanced Computing and Communication Technologies for High Performance Applications.* ACCTHPA. doi:10.1109/ACCTHPA57160.2023.10083336

N. H. R. G. P. M., S. B., Jain, & Anadkumar. (2022). E-Voting System Using Blockchain Technology. *4th International Conference on Advances in Computing, Communication Control and Networking (ICAC3N),* 2106-2111. 10.1109/ICAC3N56670.2022.10074164

Prasad, G., Jain, A. K., Jain, P., & Nagesh, H. R. (2019). A Novel Approach to Optimize the Performance of Hadoop Frameworks for Sentiment Analysis. *International Journal of Open Source Software and Processes, 10*(4), 44–59. doi:10.4018/IJOSSP.2019100103

Praveen Gujjar, J., & Prasanna Kumar, H. R. (2021). Image classification and prediction using transfer learning in colab notebook. *Global Transitions Proceedings, 2*(2), 382-385. doi:10.1016/j.gltp.2021.08.068

Praveen Gujjar, J., Prasanna Kumar, H. R., & Guru Prasad, M. S. (2023). Advanced NLP Framework for Text Processing. *6th International Conference on Information Systems and Computer Networks (ISCON),* 1-3. 10.1109/ISCON57294.2023.10112058

Singh, P., Tripathi, V., Singh, K. D., Guru Prasad, M. S., & Aditya Pai, H. (2023, April). A Task Scheduling Algorithm for Optimizing Quality of Service in Smart Healthcare System. In *International Conference on IoT, Intelligent Computing and Security: Select Proceedings of IICS 2021* (pp. 43-50). Singapore: Springer Nature Singapore. 10.1007/978-981-19-8136-4_4

Strielkina, A., Illiashenko, O., Zhydenko, M., & Uzun, D. (2018). Cybersecurity of healthcare IoT-based systems: regulation and case-oriented assessment. *2018 IEEE 9th International Conference on Dependable Systems, Services and Technologies (DESSERT),* 67–73. 10.1109/DESSERT.2018.8409101

Tully, J., Selzer, J., Phillips, J. P., O'Connor, P., & Dameff, C. (2020). Healthcare challenges in the era of cybersecurity. *Health Security, 18*(3), 228–231. doi:10.1089/hs.2019.0123 PMID:32559153

Chapter 2
Machine Learning–Based Cyber Intrusion Detection System for Internet of Medical Things Attacks in Healthcare Environments

Bhawnesh Kumar
Graphic Era University (Deemed), India

Ashwani Kumar
Shri Ram Group of Colleges, India

Harendra Singh Negi
Graphic Era University (Deemed), India

Javed Alam
Quantlase Lab, Abu Dhabi, UAE

ABSTRACT

In this chapter, the authors calculate the accuracy value of machine learning models for combined, network, bio-medical data. The result shows that random forest has the highest accuracy value 94.17% for combined and 93.19% bio-medical data. For network data, decision tree classifier provides the highest accuracy value which is 94.07% whereas decision tree regression gives the highest accuracy value: 94.62% for combined, 92.11% for bio-medical, and 94.09% for network data.

DOI: 10.4018/978-1-6684-6646-9.ch002

INTRODUCTION AND BACKGROUNDS

Sensors, the cloud, and many more advanced technologies give a new aspect to the healthcare system. Advancements in the area of wireless data collection through sensors, data storage, internet, and communication link patients who are far from healthcare professionals. Remote monitoring systems enabled the communication link between doctors and patients using various types of gadgets such as smart watches, smartphones, laptops, and many more devices. These devices are known as the internet of things (IoT). If these devices are integrated for medical purposes, then it becomes the internet of medical things (IoMT) (Razdan & Sharma, 2021). IoMT reduces the visit of the patient and medical professionals can collect the data of patients through the internet. Patient details are represented as a medical record in a digital format than paper which also knows as electronic health records (Dimitrov, 2016) (EHR). Wireless communication is used between the patient and server repository to locate the EHR details. EHR data should be secured from intruders and attacks while transmitted over communication channels through the internet. As IoMT architecture (Toghuj & Turab, 2022) shown in Fig 1 where three layers named application, network, and perception, represent the flow of data from sensors/actuators to cloud/server. These layers performed the following operations on medical data: processed, analyzed, and stored.

To do the computational statistical analysis, machine learning (ML) helped to predict intrusion detection for cyber security (Davenport & Kalakota, 2019a). The most promising technique is to manage issues of security in healthcare systems for attacks (Abouelmehdi et al., 2018). L comprises the rules and methods that can

Figure 1. IoMT architecture

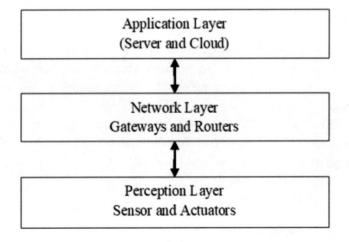

be applied to large amounts of data to find the prediction behavior and pattern of cyber security attacks. It is necessary to migrate to a run-time approach to detect intrusion when the changing patterns in network behavior (Tgavalekos et al., 2018). ML broadly splits into supervised, unsupervised, and semi-supervised learning. As supervised learning works with labeled data whereas unsupervised is used for unlabeled data and semi-supervised used for labeled and less unlabeled data (Singh et al., 2017). Supervised learning works on training and testing data (Rawat et al., 2022). ML helps to save valuable time and minimize damages due to cyber-attacks (Sarker et al., 2020). Existing classification models (Pérez-Ortiz et al., 2016) uch as Naïve Bayes (NB), decision tree (DT), support vector machine (SVM), random forest (RF), K-Nearest Neighbor (K-NN), stochastic gradient (SG), and many more are helpful to be applied on a large dataset. Some regression models (Dasgupta et al., 2011) (Negi et al., 2022) are also considered for the same dataset such as logistic, linear, lasso, ridge, decision tree, and more.

ML models can also be helpful to detect the intrusion raised when IoMT devices send their data to a server. The availability of suspicious attacks between medical devices and servers (Hireche et al., 2022) hows that noise data is appended with original data. The existence of ML models in an IoMT environment based on a detection system can help to predict cyber-attacks. The capability of ML is managing cyber-attack issues using a type of healthcare sensor (Kumar & Lee, 2011). Healthcare system has a gateway for data collection, and monitoring the network traffic need to support cyber-attacks detection system computer (Hady et al., 2020). The server is located last to store the sensed data from various sources. As the dataset has network traffic related and patient data. For predicting cyber-attacks in healthcare, various ML techniques are applied to network and patient data and evaluate the measurements metric. The following purposes are there in healthcare using ML (Davenport & Kalakota, 2019b):

- Maintaining the patient records
- Predicting the treatment procedures
- Innovating and developing the new medicines
- Providing diagnose systems
- Detecting the cyber-attacks
- Maintaining IoMT sensors

CRITICAL REVIEWS

Hady et al. (2020) implemented supervised machine learning models to network and bio data to detect the cyberattacks. Dataset prepared through sensor board named as

Enhanced Healthcare Monitoring System testbed. This board attached with universal serial bus port and window-based machine. It runs through C++ programming to sense the data from sensor board and data transferred by wi-fi connection. In between transmission attackers take place to spoof and alter the sensed data and redirect to server. After that some ML models implemented on collected network and bio data of patient to detect intrusion. ML models implemented on all data, network data and bio data separately. Find out the accuracy value of RF, SVM, KNN and artificial neural network (ANN), where ANN gives the remarkable result. In future more attacks can also be considered to enhanced the intrusion detection system for healthcare.

Karmakar et al. (2020) suggested architecture for the security of the IoMT-enabled electronic healthcare environment with an encryption-supported protocol for communication. The considered scenario is having an operation support system, provider, and resources. Requirements of security for IoMT devices are inclusive, authorization/authentication, privacy, and detection of threats. Also implemented elliptic curve cryptography protocol handles the IoMT devices.

Jain et al. (2021) suggested a security model as solution for intrusion detection based on artificial neural network for IoT enabled healthcare environment. This method predicts doubtful devices which ae based on usage of bandwidth. In this, security subsystem regularly checked the connection of all clients and machine learning is used to find out the suspicious devices. Tool used to design this model is MATLAB. Methodology of design is breaking down in to following sections: use cases of healthcare in sliced network, IoT based architecture, data flow from input to output, algorithm along with neural network. Levenberg-Marquardt and Bayesian-Regularization training functions are used for neural network. In future aspect, this paper can be extended to add data privacy module.

Ardito et al. (2021) proposed a system for cyberattack detection based on artificial techniques. There is no need for security analysts to detect anomalies and also display the attacks of a suspect to healthcare professionals. This paper focused on cases where an IoMT system has been hacked due to malicious intent of changes in the healthcare data of a patient. In the detection system of cyberattacks, architecture defined three aspects which are clinical pathway anomaly detection, explainer, and user interface (visualization). IoMT edge computing suggested a type of distributed computing that improves reliability and minimizes latency. An IoMT sensor collects various parameters of clinical. Through AI techniques in this detection system, the healthcare system can be made more secure.

Fouda et al. (2021) proposed a subclass model for intrusion detection for the internet of health things (IoHT), where deep clustering is used to prepare. The analytical tool of ML is used to improve the security of IoHT and also gives an improvement in case of detection rate, reducing the false negatives. For future work, this model can also be implemented on large datasets without affecting performance.

Chuwu et al. (2021) applied the ML techniques to detect malicious behavior or attack in IoT healthcare networks and worked for imbalanced data. This work has a 2-phase where the first is for network protocol and the second is based on long short-term memory. The proposed work has four stages preprocess, categorization of protocol, selection of features, and anomaly detection. For detection, the accuracy of long short-term memory (LSTM) is 97.06%, 94.85% is for precision, recall value is 97.42% with the comparison of SVM and convolutional neural network (CNN).

Vaiyapuri et al. (2021) explained system literature review on security concerns for IoMT-enabled smart healthcare systems. Parameters focused on data transmission, authentication, confidentiality, access control, and privacy-preserving. Also, explain the strengths and weaknesses of some research papers. A weakness of one of them is ML techniques are not supported in a defined system. The future section mentioned that an efficient and lightweight detection system should be developed for the IoMT-enabled healthcare system.

Thomas and Bhat (2021) gives a survey paper between 2014 and 2021 that deals with an intrusion detection system for IoT security. Various ML supervised and supervised techniques that follow naïve Bayes, K-NN, decision tree, support vector machine, random forest, K-means and many more can be helpful to detect intrusions. Research gaps were identified which are a lack of accuracy and the need to reduce the complexity. Deep learning can also be helpful to improve the detection the intrusion systems.

Akshay Kumaar et al. (2022) proposed a deep learning-based hybrid framework to identify the intrusions attacks. This system is named as ImmuneNet. New cyber-attacks were found to protect patient data. As neural network model has achieved 99.2% accuracy level. In the future, a self-supervised learning approach can be based on neural networks to detect new attacks.

Kayode Saheed et al. (2022) applied supervised learning to detect attacks on IoT networks. Initially, min-max of normalization was used, and later on dimension reduction through principal component analysis. Finally, various types of ML techniques are implemented on the given dataset. To train the dataset, KNN, SVM, extreme gradient boosting (XGBoost), naïve Bayes, and many more classifiers were used. The proposed model gives an accuracy 99.99%. In the future, an ensemble model can also be used to detect IoT attacks in a healthcare environment.

Si-Ahmed et al. (2022) gives a comprehensive survey to detect IoMT attacks using ML for security purposes. Presented a 3-layers model of IoMT to secure the healthcare system (data collection, transmission, and storage level). At each layer which types of ML techniques are applicable. As kinds of threats can decrease the performance of IoMT based secure model which affects the working procedure of medical staff. Identify the merits, demerits, and methodology for the corresponding healthcare system.

Hireche et al. (2022) proposed a study on various security techniques which are dedicated to the healthcare environment. In IoMT architecture, each layer specifies the attacks such as the perception layer having side channels, tampering devices, tag cloning, and sensor tracking. In network layer attacks are eavesdropping, replay, denial of services (DoS), sinkhole, sniffing, and many more. At the application layer, attacks are listed as brute force, structured query language (SQL) injection, account hijacking, and ransomware. Various models are mentioned in this paper such as blockchain, authentication, and machine learning models. This paper focused on the current security and privacy in IoMT.

As many research papers are considered to review the existing directions of IDS for IoMT-based healthcare systems. ML-based techniques were applied to different parameters to find out the accuracy value which is shown in Table I.

MACHINE LEARNING MODELS

Artificial intelligence and machine learning models are available to make the advanced computer system. This is also an open space for an organization can leverage advancement to drive output and make an impact on the bottom line(Javaid et al., 2022). The healthcare environment includes the development of new advanced systems for medical purposes. Various ML-supervised models are considered for this chapter to predict the attacks on healthcare systems shown in Figure 2.

K-NN is used for classification-based ML model and classified the data points as per neighbors (Mucherino et al., 2009). The measurement of classification is based on the similarity of the earlier stored data points. It is simple to implement, learn for no-linear decision boundaries, no training time, and evolves new data and distance metrics. Assume the equality of all features, for large datasets prediction complexity, is high and dimension is high then outliers can have a high impact. Naïve Bayes (Xu, 2018) used the Bayes rule for strong, this algorithm not used a single algorithm it combines many. Where shared a common principle which is every pair of features should be classified independently of each other. Two assumptions are considered independent and equal to contribute to the outcome. Commonly used for recommendation systems, spam filtering, sentiment analysis, and many more. The requirement of predictor should be independent which is a lack of this model. A decision tree is used for both classification and regression types of problems. It has two node decisions and a leaf node where the decision node is used for decision whereas the leaf is used for output. It is used for the decision-related problem, and can also think of all possible outcomes and fewer requirements for the data cleaning process. Due to having more layers, it becomes complex. As class labels increased the complexity of this algorithm may also increase. Random forest (Breiman, 2001)

Table 1. Machine learning techniques-based solutions for IDS for IoMT-based healthcare system

Sr.no	Author	Purpose	Technique Used	Accuracy	
1.	Thamilarasu et al. (2020)	Design a IDS for network connected devices	Mobile agent-based intrusion detection system	99.6(network) and 98.2% (device level)	
2.	Newaz et al. (2020)	New IDS for attacks to medical devices	Proposed HEKA	98.4%	
3.	Hady et al. (2020)	Comparison study on IDS for Healthcare.	Random Forest, KNN, SVM, ANN	For combined 91.45%(RF), 87.48%(KNN), 82.37%(SVM) and 93.42%(ANN).	
4.	Radoglou-Grammatikis et al. (2021)	Self-learning approach for IDS in healthcare	DT NB SVM RF Multi-layer perceptron (MLP) Dense Deep Neural network (DNN) Relu Dense DNN tanh	**HTTP** 96.44% 72.88% 89.07% 92.29% 90.47% 90.90% 94.07%	**TCP** 83.33% 71.98% 84.10% 94.45% 81.79% 88.35% 94.07%
5.	Chuwu et al. (2021)	Detection of IoT attacks using ML in healthcare	LSTM, SVM, CNN	LSTM accuracy is 97.06% and SVM is 92.45% accurate. 91.59% accuracy for CNN.	
6.	Subasi et al. (2021)	Detection of intrusion in smart healthcare	Bagging with random forest	97.67%	
7.	Thanh Nguyen et al. (2021)	Multimodal fusion framework based on deep learning for IDS in healthcare data	decision-based fusion model	99.21%	
8.	Fouda et al. (2021)	IDS for IoHT using deep subclasses dispersion	Gaussian, Support Vector Data Description, One-class Support Vector Machine, Mahalanobis One-class Support Vector Machine, One-Class-Neural Network, Subclass dispersion one class SVM	(5-fold) 84.36% 94.12% 92.95% 92.74% 76.08% 96.91%	
9.	Hussain et al. (2021)	Framework for malicious traffic Detection in IoT Healthcare Environment	NB KNN RF Adaboost (AB) Logistic Regression (Log R) DT	99.70% 99.68% 99.79% 99.44% 90.35% 99.79%	

continued on following page

Table 1. Continued

Sr.no	Author	Purpose	Technique Used	Accuracy
10.	Akshay Kumaar et al. (2022)	Framework for IDS using deep learning for healthcare	ImmuneNet XGBoost Random Forest Decision trees Logistics Regression	99.19% 9910% 98.21% 97.66% 92.87%
11.	Kayode Saheed et al. (2022)	ML based IDS.	XGBoost Cat Boost KNN SVM Quadratic Discriminant Analysis (QDA) NB	99.99% 99.99% 99.98% 99.98% 99.97% 97.14%
12.	Sengan et al. (2022)	DoS detection system by ML algorithm	Dynamic Secure aware Routing by Machine Learning	98.19%

Figure 2. ML models

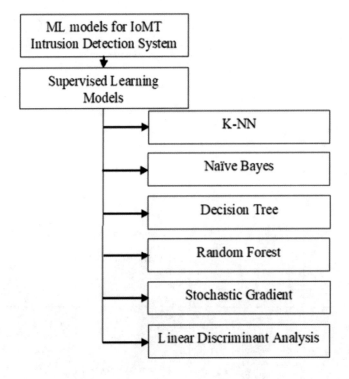

model is based on the ensemble method which combines bagging and boosting. Where bagging selects a random sample from the dataset and row sampling with replacement is known as bootstrap. The following features are considered for random forest stability, train and test, dimensionality, diversity, and parallelization. The stochastic gradient model (Bottou, 2012) is used to find the parameters for the best fit between actual and predicted outcomes. It is an iterative mathematical optimization method and it is also optimized internally to get model parameters. It has three types such as batch, and stochastic mini-batch. Stochastic is a word that is co-related with a random probability. Linear discriminant analysis (LDA) is used to reduce the dimensions to solve the 2-class classification problems. Using a single feature when we classify then it may show overlapping. To solve the overlapping we have to separate them efficiently into 2-classes with multiple features. LDA is used for face detection, customer identification, medical, decision making, and robots. Quadratic and flexible both are two extensions of LDA. Regression models are used to find out the relationship between target and predictor variables. For future prediction, regression models are helpful such as sales prediction, weather prediction, market trends and many more (Doan & Kalita, 2015).

PERFORMANCE EVALUATION AND RESULT ANALYSIS

Evaluate the performance of various machine learning models implemented on network and medical datasets. Dataset is downloaded from https://www.cse.wustl.edu/~jain/ehms/index.html and is also referred to by Hardy (Hady et al., 2020). In this dataset, two groups are there one is related to network data and another group is related to bio-medical data. In network data, 27 attributes are there whereas in bio-medical, 8 attributes and 1 attribute is for target value. Types of attacks considered spoofing, data alteration, and dataset splits into a 70:30 ratio for train and test sets. Experimental purpose work done in Python on a dell laptop with the configuration of processor 11th Gen Intel(R) Core (TM) i5-11320H @ 3.20GHz 2.50 GHz, RAM is 16 GB and OS is windows 11. Machine learning models are KNN, NB, DT, RF, SG, and LDA considered for implementation shown in Figure 3. Performance parameter is accuracy calculated for each model on network data, bio-medical data, and combined.

The random forest has the highest accuracy value 94.17% for combined and 93.19% for bio-medical data. For network data, the decision tree classifier provides the highest accuracy value which is 94.07%. Regression models also considered finding the accuracy value which is logistic, linear, lasso, ridge, and decision tree shown in Figure 4. Decision tree regression gives the highest accuracy value i.e., 94.62% for combined, 92.11% for bio-medical, and 94.09% for network data. As various ML models are implemented to find out the accuracy value to predict cyber-attacks. These results have shown that to design the health monitoring system, ML

Figure 3. Accuracy of classifier

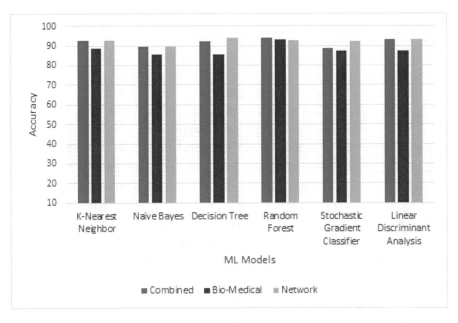

Figure 4. Accuracy of regression

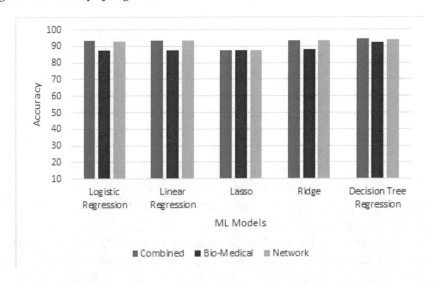

models play a vital role to have a cyber-attack detection system. Results prove that the performance of the detection system based on the ML models applied and random forest and decision tree both are best suited for healthcare systems.

RESEARCH DIRECTIONS

- More attacks can also be considered to enhance the intrusion detection system for healthcare (Hady et al., 2020).
- Extended to add data privacy module (Jain et al., 2021).
- An incremental IoHT model can also be developed to overcome the limitations of being a batch-learning model. This model can also be implemented on large datasets without affecting performance (Fouda et al., 2021).
- An efficient and lightweight detection system should be developed for IoMT-enabled healthcare systems (Vaiyapuri et al., 2021).
- Research gaps were identified which are a lack of accuracy and the need to reduce the complexity. Deep learning can also be helpful to improve the detection the intrusion systems (Thomas & Bhat, 2021).
- Self-supervised learning approach, which can be based on the neural network to detect new attacks (Akshay Kumaar et al., 2022).
- The ensemble model can also be used to detect IoT attacks in the healthcare environment (Kayode Saheed et al., 2022).
- Need of developing of IoT based healthcare system which should be a more robust context-aware security solution (Hussain et al., 2021).
- Integration of advanced IDS system with existing safeguard mechanisms (Chuwu et al., 2021).

CONCLUSION

Machine learning models help predict the cyber-attacks in IoMT healthcare environment. Advancement in the healthcare field needs to develop the IoMT sensor devices-based system to collect patient details remotely through the internet. As collected data is used to predict the treatment plan for new coming patients. As patient data is transferred on the network then suspicious attacks are done by intruders that add or alter the patient details. This may lead to a decrease in the diagnosis system performance which may also impact patient treatment planning. To design IDS, ML gives the direction to find out the cyber-attacks on healthcare data. Various types of ML classification and regression models are implemented on network-related data as well as on patient-related data. Calculate the accuracy value of each implemented model for combined, network, and bio-medical data. The random forest has the highest accuracy value 94.17% for combined and 93.19% for bio-medical data. For network data, the decision tree classifier provides the highest accuracy value which is 94.07%. Decision tree regression gives the highest accuracy value i.e., 94.62% for combined, 92.11% for bio-medical, and 94.09% for network data. In the future, deep learning, neural network, and conventional neural network-based models can also be implemented to design the detection system for cyber-attacks in a healthcare environment.

REFERENCES

Abouelmehdi, K., Beni-Hessane, A., & Khaloufi, H. (2018). Big healthcare data: Preserving security and privacy. *Journal of Big Data*, 5(1), 1. Advance online publication. doi:10.118640537-017-0110-7

Akshay Kumaar, M., Samiayya, D., Vincent, P. M. D. R., Srinivasan, K., Chang, C. Y., & Ganesh, H. (2022). A Hybrid Framework for Intrusion Detection in Healthcare Systems Using Deep Learning. *Frontiers in Public Health*, 9, 824898. Advance online publication. doi:10.3389/fpubh.2021.824898 PMID:35096763

Ardito, C., di Noia, T., di Sciascio, E., Lofù, D., Pazienza, A., & Vitulano, F. (2021). An Artificial Intelligence Cyberattack Detection System to Improve Threat Reaction in e-Health. *Italian Conference on Cybersecurity*. http://ceur-ws.org

Bottou, L. (2012). Stochastic Gradient Descent Tricks. In Neural Networks: Tricks of the Trade (pp. 421–436). doi:10.1007/978-3-642-35289-8_25

Breiman, L. (2001). Random Forests. *Machine Learning*, 45(1), 5–32. doi:10.1023/A:1010933404324

Chuwu, L., Chen, C.-M., Cai, Z.-X., Hsu, M. H., & Juang, W.-C. (2021). Machine learning-based detection of internet of thing attacks in healthcare environments. *IT in Industry, 9*(2).

Dasgupta, A., Sun, Y., König, I. R., Bailey-Wilson, J. E., & Malley, J. D. (2011). Brief review of regression-based and machine learning methods in genetic epidemiology: The Genetic Analysis Workshop 17 experience. *Genetic Epidemiology*, 35(S1), S5–S11. doi:10.1002/gepi.20642 PMID:22128059

Davenport, T., & Kalakota, R. (2019). The potential for artificial intelligence in healthcare. *Future Healthcare Journal*, 6(2), 94–102. doi:10.7861/futurehosp.6-2-94 PMID:31363513

Dimitrov, D. v. (2016). Medical internet of things and big data in healthcare. In Healthcare Informatics Research (Vol. 22, Issue 3, pp. 156–163). Korean Society of Medical Informatics. doi:10.4258/hir.2016.22.3.156

Doan, T., & Kalita, J. (2015). Selecting Machine Learning Algorithms Using Regression Models. *2015 IEEE International Conference on Data Mining Workshop (ICDMW)*, 1498–1505. 10.1109/ICDMW.2015.43

FoudaM.KsantiniR.ElmedanyW. (2021). A Novel Intrusion Detection System for Internet of Healthcare Things Based on Deep Subclasses Dispersion Information. TechRxiv. *Powered by IEEE*. doi:10.36227/techrxiv.19292444.v1

Hady, A. A., Ghubaish, A., Salman, T., Unal, D., & Jain, R. (2020). Intrusion Detection System for Healthcare Systems Using Medical and Network Data: A Comparison Study. *IEEE Access : Practical Innovations, Open Solutions*, 8, 106576–106584. doi:10.1109/ACCESS.2020.3000421

Hireche, R., Mansouri, H., & Pathan, A.-S. K. (2022). Security and Privacy Management in Internet of Medical Things (IoMT): A Synthesis. *Journal of Cybersecurity and Privacy*, 2(3), 640–661. doi:10.3390/jcp2030033

Hussain, F., Abbas, S. G., Shah, G. A., Pires, I. M., Fayyaz, U. U., Shahzad, F., Garcia, N. M., & Zdravevski, E. (2021). A framework for malicious traffic detection in iot healthcare environment. *Sensors (Basel)*, 21(9), 3025. Advance online publication. doi:10.339021093025 PMID:33925813

Jain, A., Singh, T., & Sharma, S. K. (2021). Security as a solution: An intrusion detection system using a neural network for IoT enabled healthcare ecosystem. *Interdisciplinary Journal of Information, Knowledge, and Management*, 16, 331–369. doi:10.28945/4838

Javaid, M., Haleem, A., Pratap Singh, R., Suman, R., & Rab, S. (2022). Significance of machine learning in healthcare: Features, pillars and applications. *International Journal of Intelligent Networks*, 3, 58–73. doi:10.1016/j.ijin.2022.05.002

Karmakar, K. K., Varadharajan, V., Tupakula, U., Nepal, S., & Thapa, C. (2020). Towards a Security Enhanced Virtualised Network Infrastructure for Internet of Medical Things (IoMT). *IEEE International Conference on Network Softwarization (NetSoft)*, 257–261. 10.1109/NetSoft48620.2020.9165387

Kayode Saheed, Y., Idris Abiodun, A., Misra, S., Kristiansen Holone, M., & Colomo-Palacios, R. (2022). A machine learning-based intrusion detection for detecting internet of things network attacks. *Alexandria Engineering Journal*, 61(12), 9395–9409. doi:10.1016/j.aej.2022.02.063

Kumar, P., & Lee, H.-J. (2011). Security Issues in Healthcare Applications Using Wireless Medical Sensor Networks: A Survey. *Sensors (Basel)*, 12(1), 55–91. doi:10.3390120100055 PMID:22368458

Mucherino, A., Papajorgji, P. J., & Pardalos, P. M. (2009). k-Nearest Neighbor Classification. In Springer Optimization and Its Applications (pp. 83–106). doi:10.1007/978-0-387-88615-2_4

Negi, H. S., Dimri, S. C., Kumar, B., & Singh, A. (2022). Crop Prediction Based on Soil Properties using Machine Learning for Smart Farming. *2022 International Conference on Computational Intelligence and Sustainable Engineering Solutions (CISES)*, 366–370. 10.1109/CISES54857.2022.9844274

Newaz, A. I., Sikder, A. K., Babun, L., & Uluagac, A. S. (2020). HEKA: A Novel Intrusion Detection System for Attacks to Personal Medical Devices. *2020 IEEE Conference on Communications and Network Security (CNS)*, 1–9. 10.1109/CNS48642.2020.9162311

Pérez-Ortiz, M., Jiménez-Fernández, S., Gutiérrez, P. A., Alexandre, E., Hervás-Martínez, C., & Salcedo-Sanz, S. (2016). A review of classification problems and algorithms in renewable energy applications. In Energies (Vol. 9, Issue 8). MDPI AG. doi:10.3390/en9080607

Radoglou-Grammatikis, P., Sarigiannidis, P., Efstathopoulos, G., Lagkas, T., Fragulis, G., & Sarigiannidis, A. (2021, June 1). A Self-Learning Approach for Detecting Intrusions in Healthcare Systems. *IEEE International Conference on Communications*. 10.1109/ICC42927.2021.9500354

Rawat, V., Gulati, K., Kaur, U., Seth, J. K., Solanki, V., Venkatesh, A. N., Singh, D. P., Singh, N., & Loganathan, M. (2022). A Supervised Learning Identification System for Prognosis of Breast Cancer. *Mathematical Problems in Engineering*, *2022*, 1–8. doi:10.1155/2022/7459455

Razdan, S., & Sharma, S. (2021). Internet of Medical Things (IoMT): Overview, Emerging Technologies, and Case Studies. In IETE Technical Review (Institution of Electronics and Telecommunication Engineers, India). Taylor and Francis Ltd. doi:10.1080/02564602.2021.1927863

Sarker, I. H., Kayes, A. S. M., Badsha, S., Alqahtani, H., Watters, P., & Ng, A. (2020). Cybersecurity data science: An overview from machine learning perspective. *Journal of Big Data*, *7*(1), 41. Advance online publication. doi:10.118640537-020-00318-5

Sengan, S., Khalaf, O. I., Vidya Sagar, P., Sharma, D. K., Arokia Jesu Prabhu, L., & Hamad, A. A. (2022). Secured and Privacy-Based IDS for Healthcare Systems on E-Medical Data Using Machine Learning Approach. *International Journal of Reliable and Quality E-Healthcare*, *11*(3), 1–11. doi:10.4018/IJRQEH.289175

Si-AhmedA.Al-GaradiM. A.BoustiaN. (2022). Survey of Machine Learning Based Intrusion Detection Methods for Internet of Medical Things. *ArXiv Preprint*. https://arxiv.org/abs/2202.09657

Singh, N., Singh, D. P., & Pant, B. (2017). A Comprehensive Study of Big Data Machine Learning Approaches and Challenges. *2017 International Conference on Next Generation Computing and Information Systems (ICNGCIS)*, 80–85. 10.1109/ICNGCIS.2017.14

Subasi, A., Algebsani, S., Alghamdi, W., Kremic, E., Almaasrani, J., & Abdulaziz, N. (2021). Intrusion Detection in Smart Healthcare Using Bagging Ensemble Classifier. In CMBEBIH 2021 (pp. 164–171). doi:10.1007/978-3-030-73909-6_18

Tgavalekos, K., Namayanja, J. M., & Alhassan, R. (2018). Characterization of network behavior to detect changes. *Proceedings of the Workshop Program of the 19th International Conference on Distributed Computing and Networking*, 1–6. 10.1145/3170521.3170523

Thamilarasu, G., Odesile, A., & Hoang, A. (2020). An Intrusion Detection System for Internet of Medical Things. *IEEE Access : Practical Innovations, Open Solutions*, 8, 181560–181576. doi:10.1109/ACCESS.2020.3026260

Thanh Nguyen, P., Dang Bich Huynh, V., Dang Vo, K., Thanh Phan, P., Elhoseny, M., & Le, D.-N. (2021). Deep Learning based Optimal Multimodal Fusion Framework for Intrusion Detection Systems for Healthcare Data. *Computers, Materials & Continua*, 66(3), 2555–2571. doi:10.32604/cmc.2021.012941

Thomas, L., & Bhat, S. (2021). Machine Learning and Deep Learning Techniques for IoT-based Intrusion Detection Systems: A Literature Review. *International Journal of Management, Technology, and Social Sciences,* 6(2), 296–314. doi:10.5281/zenodo.5814702

Toghuj, W., & Turab, N. (2022). A survey on security threats in the internet of medical things (IoMT). *Journal of Theoretical and Applied Information Technology*, 100(10). www.jatit.org

Vaiyapuri, T., Binbusayyis, A., & Varadarajan, V. (2021). Security, Privacy and Trust in IoMT Enabled Smart Healthcare System: A Systematic Review of Current and Future Trends. *IJACSA). International Journal of Advanced Computer Science and Applications*, 12(2), 731–737. doi:10.14569/IJACSA.2021.0120291

Xu, S. (2018). Baycsian Naïve Bayes classifiers to text classification. *Journal of Information Science*, 44(1), 48–59. doi:10.1177/0165551516677946

Chapter 3
Blockchain–Enabled Smart Healthcare Systems Using IoT

Abhishek Kumar
School of Computer and Systems Sciences, Jawaharlal Nehru University, India

Karan Singh
School of Computer and Systems Sciences, Jawaharlal Nehru University, India

ABSTRACT

A healthcare system is the medical platform through which patients get better treatment. Several hospitals and doctors are linked together through this platform in a hierarchy and treat the patient easily. In view of the COVID-19 pandemic, it is a very challenging task to treat the patients physically; therefore, there is a need to redevelop the healthcare system to fulfill the modern demand. The state of the art of this scheme is to provide remote treatment facilities and build a secure online system. Blockchain technology combined with IoT provides the solution through its vital features of transparency, immutability, decentralization, and trust-less environment. IoT devices capture the patient health status and process it and send to blockchain; therefore, information sharing between devices, hospitals, and doctors are at risk and need to provide security. Using key management scheme in smart contract to ensure integrity of data, this scheme provides better treatment at cheap cost as well as efficiency and security compared to traditional healthcare systems.

INTRODUCTION

Healthcare system is the common platform to provide better treatment facility to the patient. Through this common platform authority can manage the patient

DOI: 10.4018/978-1-6684-6646-9.ch003

record and provide treatment facility. In this system many hospital are connected in a hierarchy and when need to refer the patient for treatment, authority can share the stored patient treatment information to another hospital for better treatment even store information for further treatment. Due to huge population growth the health sector is suffered from modern problem create a socio economic problem. Even less number of hospital and limited resource cause many problems to keep proper functioning of healthcare system and still many ruler areas contain no hospital facility (Budida et al., 2017). In view of covid pandemic doctor treat the patient in online mode to keep safe the other people from pandemic and patient has no need to came hospital while patient has not severe condition and it is very challenging task to doctor treat the patient physically therefore future trend using Blockchain and IoT device can resolve these issue. Doctor can remotely access the patient health status with the help of IoT device capture the data from patient body and this will also helpful to remote area people (Chamola et al., 2020). While online mode of treatment the record of patient is most important and need to store long period of time, even many hospital are connected to common platform if needed for better treatment doctor can share the patient information to other place, IoT device time to time keep record the patient health status like temperature, heartbeat, oxygen level, blood pressure, etc. and update the patient record automatically leads to generate huge data and need to proper faster storage and maintenance therefore security and transparency of data are one of aspect (De Aguiar et al., 2020). In traditional system many serious problems like centralized database used to maintain the record, no proper authentication mechanisms is available for participating entity, less number of transaction, and suffer from many cryptographic attack. The Blockchain technology provides the solution of above mention problem through its features in term of transparency, decentralization, immutable and trust less environment. When multiple party seemingly belonging across the world and need to share data, transfer value without trusting each other this was major problem in the modern world and it is happily resolve with Blockchain technology (Dwivedi et al., 2021). Blockchain is the share ledger which store the data whereas Decentralized feature support fault tolerance because data is not store at single point. Immutable feature ensure that no one can change the single character store inside. Every participating entity can view the transaction at any point of time to make system transparent. IoT is the light computing device which is capturing the data, proses it and deliver over internet therefore IoT make system smarter and reduce human effort (Lockl et al., 2020). Using IoT device to make more smart healthcare system and getting more reliable and continent treatment facility. The state of the art of this chapter is we present a Blockchain based secure information sharing in smart health care system with smart contract and consensus mechanism. The key management technique ensures that only authorized entity be a part of existing network. Blockchain based key distribution among all participating entity using smart contract to provide security of data with the help of existing block and transaction validation protocol and try to upgrade the security of the system (Dwivedi et al., 2020).

BACKGROUND

Blockchain Overview

The history of blockchain, blockchain technology invented first time in 1991 by the two popular research scientist Stuart Haber and W. Scott Stornetta, They try to store the time stamp document using new concept cryptographically secure chain of block. In 1992, blockchain technology get more efficient when markle trees were concept incorporated and allow multiple document store in one block. It is helpful in creating secure chain of block. In 2004 computer scientist Hal Finney introduced new system called Reusable Proof of work a Backbone of digital cash. Further, Blockchain get famous when most popular cryptocurrency bitcoin came into picture. Bitcoin is a public blockchain develop by Satoshi Nakamoto in 2008. It is decentralized peer-to-peer electronic transfer i.e. without involvement of third party like bank and it is based on proof-of-work consensus method for tracking and verification of transaction and each transaction is protected through digital signature (Zou et al., 2020).

In simple word, blockchain is a shared database, which contain ledger of transaction i.e. record of transaction like bank but not like centralized bank. In blockchain system every device has a copy of ledger and it might be verify each other accounts. Every connected device with a copy of ledger is called namely "Node". Due to its vital features like distributed, decentralized given in Figure 1, immutable, transparent, trust-less and anonymity makes it's more secure and reduces human efforts toward manual work (Kouhizadeh et al., 2018). Its decentralized feature provide fault tolerance, immutable feature means transaction or file record can't be change even single latter changing means entire blockchain violations. Transparent means every entity involve in system can keep track of transaction any time anywhere. Trust less means every one share the record without trust because no third party involve in between the transaction and anonymity means hide the sender or receiver personal information. So finally blockchain is a technology in which block are connected through a cryptographic link. Blockchain is capable to solving the problem like tempering the product, fraud, delay, supply chain system, smart agriculture system, cryptocurrency and it is more famous when cryptocurrency bitcoin came in market.

Figure 1. Node connectivity type network

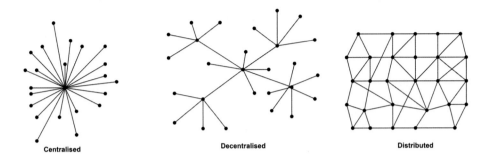

Centralised   Decentralised   Distributed

Major Role of Blockchain

When multiple party seemingly belonging across the world and need to share data, transfer value without trusting each other this was major problem in the modern world and it is happily resolve with blockchain technology. The financial world define the trust is the counterparty risk therefore Blockchain entirely remove the counterparty risk with the revolutionary system of mathematics, cryptography and peer-to-peer networking. However blockchain eliminate the risk of trust that affect another database with the help of these three term (Wüst et al., 2018).

- **Full Decentralization:** Reading/Writing is fully decentralized and secure i.e. not control under single or group of person.
- **Extreme Fault Tolerance:** Capability system to handle corrupt data.
- **Independent Verification:** Transaction can verified by any node, without third party.

Structure of Blockchain

Figure 2 given the structure of blockchain which contain block index unique number to identify block, nonce a random number depend on difficulty level, data store in block, previous hash used to link block and first block hash is entire 256 bit is zero called genesis block which is indicate the starting block of chain, and current hash.

Block

It contain list of transaction which is mined together therefore it is a place where information stored and encrypted through cryptographic function. Block identified

Figure 2. General view of block in blockchain

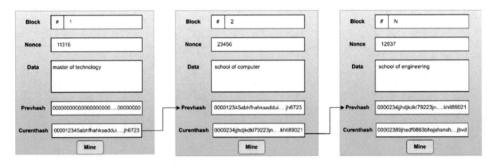

by long number including encrypt transaction information from previous block and new transaction information.

The network in the system is must verify the block and its conation data before creation of new block. Every block in the blockchain network is connected through a high secure cryptographic link. The first block of blockchain is called genesis block because of previous hash of genesis block is 0 (Tosh et al., 2017). There are some basic field involve in block is as follows.

Magic Number: In case of cryptocurrency, it is a number contains specific value that is used to identify a block is part of the network.

Block Size: It is a value setting to size of block to writing limited amount of information on the block.

Block Header: It contain information about the block.

Transaction Counter: A kind of number that identify how many transaction stored in the block.

Transaction: A list of all record in the form of transaction in a block.

Version: The cryptocurrency version used in case of cryptocurrency blockchain.

Time: A timestamp inside block in the blockchain.

Bits: It is a difficulty level current hash, signifying the difficulty in the solving the nonce.

Hash Markle Root: The current block hash of transaction in the markle tree.

Nonce: It is kind of special number used once to find the solution of the blockchain problem and also helpful in define the transaction number for an account or address.

Previous Hash: It is 256 bit encrypted number knows as hash based on previous blocks header.

Current Hash: It is a 256 bit or 64 digit encrypted number based on addition of hash of nonce, data, current hash.

Mine: Process of finding the solution of problem like find the hash contain starting with four zero.

Hash: It is fixed length unique string to identify a piece of data calculated based on available cryptographic hash function (SHA-256, keccak-256).

Classification of Blockchain

Basically blockchain is categorized on the basis of consensus process is two types namely permissionless and permissioned. Figure 3 given the crystal idea of these blockchain. Public blockchain is fully permissionless where private and consortium are fully permissioned and hybrid are combination of both.

In permissionless, it is open network allow anyone to interaction with consensus validation and full decentralized also called public, Trust less. There are many key attribute which is full transparent, development in open source, mostly anonymous, privacy depend on technological limitation, not control authority and involve digital assets. These attribute helpful to decide which type of blockchain i prefer to needed work. There is some biggest benefit in term of broader decentralization, highly transparent, censorship resistant and security resilience. It has also a market traction like P2P, B2C and government to citizens. Overall there are neither restrictions, and participation is also not controlled under admin. Any one participate in the consensus network to validate the data. Neither any administrator allow the user to getting permission to any kind of modification. Therefore permissionless blockchain is entirely decentralized blockchain platform across unknown parties (Peng et al., 2021).

In permissioned, it is a closed network with limited decentralize and designated parties for participation in consensus validation of network therefore it is also called as Private, Permissioned Sandbox. There are some key point which is controlled transparency, development by private entities, Non anonymous, privacy based on governance decision, not single authority, may or may not involve digital assets. The key point help us to choose relevant blockchain according to our requirement. Permission blockchain has many benefit like incremental decentralization, strong privacy, customize, faster and Scalable. This blockchain have market transaction B2B, B2C and Government organization. However very few user permissioned by administrator to access the distributed ledger. Due to limitation user grant to do certain action. If admin not allowed anyone, then no one permit to access it publicly. The greatest advantage of this model is to user accessing the ledger are limited, any kind of modification in the ledger can be easily tracked and identified the user. It is a kind of addition layer of security in the blockchain. Permission blockchain used in business operation mainly where data security is more important. It will be used in supply chains, creating contract, and payment verification (Liu et al., 2019).

Public Blockchain: Public blockchain grant every nodes of the network have to identical rights to access the blockchain, create new block of data, and validate block of data in the network so public blockchain is complete decentralized in nature.

Figure 3. Classification of blockchain

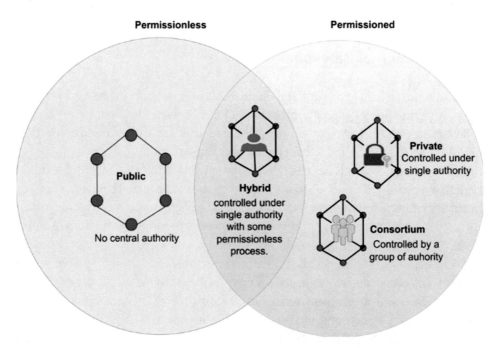

Cryptocurrency like Bitcoin, Ethereum, Litecoin, primarily used public blockchain for exchanging and mining cryptocurrency. The node "mine" means by creating block based on transactions requested on the system by solving cryptographic puzzle or cryptographic equation. Those node who solve the puzzle with effort of hard work getting reward in term of cryptocurrency (Norman et al., 2018).

Private Blockchain: Private Blockchain has single control authority and the central authority decide to who can be a node. The central authority do not allow to every node have same rights to perform functions. It is partially decentralize because user access is restricted. Business-to-business (B2B) virtual currency exchange network like Ripple and Hyperledger is universal open source are popular example of private block. Compare to public blockchain have longer validation time for new data where as private blockchain has more vulnerable to fraud and bad actors (Dhakal et al., 2019).

Consortium Blockchain: It is govern by group of entity, rather than one entity in case of private blockchain. So there is higher decentralization than private blockchain result leads to high level of security. It offers new kind of it the block to add the established structure and send information instead of initial from scratch. This technique help system to find resolution and save time based on development cost. For the financial services a poplar set of consortium blockchain in industry and beyond has been develop by the enterprise software firm R3. CargoSmart has been developed the Global shipping Business Network consortium in the supply chain. The development of research 74% of system are prefer consortium as a blockchain (Meng et al., 2021).

Hybrid Blockchain: A hybrid blockchain is a special kind of blockchain technology that combines elements of both private and public blockchains and aims to use the best features of both types of blockchains. Transactions and data are made private but can still be validated as necessary, for as by granting access via a smart contract. Although retained inside the network, private information can still be verified. IBM food trust an example of hybrid blockchain to improve efficiency throughout the whole food supply chain (Zhu et al., 2019).

Blockchain Version

There are different version given in Figure 4 where blockchain version such as version 1.0 for currency, version 2.0 for smart contract, and version 3.0 for decentralized application.

Blockchain Version 1.0: Is dedicated especially for currency. The idea behind to creating digital money with the help of solving difficult computational puzzle through block mining process was invented in 2005 by Hal Finney. He introduced first time cryptocurrency i.e. implementation of distributed ledger. This ledger permit financial transaction based on blockchain technology to execute Bitcoin.

Blockchain Version 2.0: With smart contract concept came in picture because the mining process take heavy wasting of energy it will cause lack of scalability in network.

Smart contract is a script or piece of code written in high level programming language which is execute inside blockchain automatically. So mining concept eliminate by smart contract. Ethereum blockchain get introduced here which provide platform where we can build distributed application and enhance high security with highest daily transaction.

Blockchain Version 3.0: Especially dedicated to decentralized application which is has decentralized communication and storage facility. The backend code run

Figure 4. Blockchain version

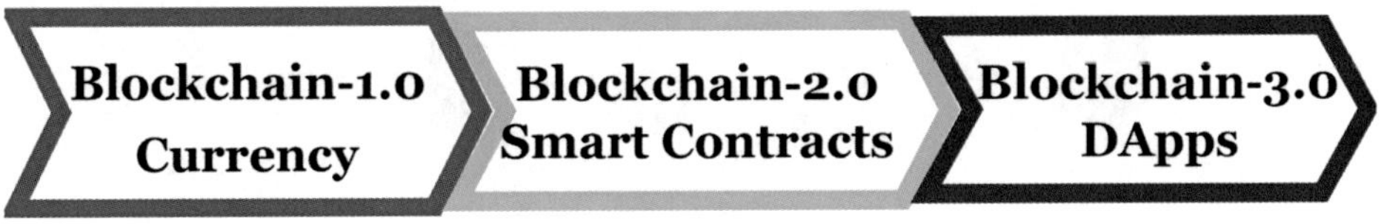

inside decentralized peer-to-peer node. DApp might have frontend code hosted on decentralized storage like Ethereum Swarm and user interfaces written any language which make possible to call backend code (Khan et al., 2019).

Working Principle of Blockchain

Let user X want to send some money like crypto value to user Y, given in Figure 5 then X send a transaction request where transaction create in one of block of blockchain after that these block is send to every node of the network. With the help of validation algorithm transaction validate by validator node. After successful validation new block is created and every node is update the latest copy of ledger. Those node who are hard working to validating the transaction through "mining" process getting some reward. Finally new block is added to the existing blockchain and money is successfully transferred to user Y (Madaan et al., 2020).

Application of Blockchain

Money Transfer: Money transfer through blockchain is cost reduction and faster compare to traditional transfer services. It will enhance the transaction rate per day.

This is particularly true with cross border transaction which also are frequently delayed and costly.

Financial Exchange: Many organization invented decentralized cryptocurrency exchange. With the help of blockchain exchange permit faster and low expansive

Figure 5. Workflow architecture of blockchain

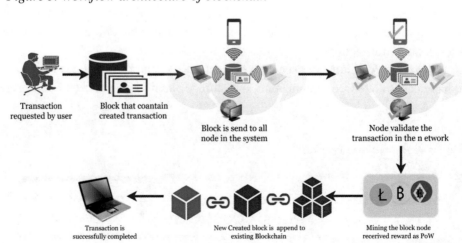

transactions. In decentralized system doesn't need to investor deposited assets with centralized authority i.e. they maintain more security (Berentsen et al., 2019).

Lending: It is used blockchain to implement collateralized loans using smart contract. Smart contract allow automatically trigger certain thing like payment, margin call, full repayment of the loan. Result leads to fastest processing of loan with cheap cost.

Insurance: Blockchain provide more transparency for customers and insurance company using smart contract. Smart contract create a kind of contract between user and company in term of record like auto premium payment, bond, terms and condition, and identity. When bond period end then money automatically credit to beneficiaries account. It will help to speed up the process and keep transparent to maintain integrity.

Real Estate: In real state lot of paper work done and very much overhead the system to keep record safe, verify financial information, ownership and then send deeds and titles to new owners. Blockchain provide more security and transferring ownership that will help to speed up the transaction, reduce paper work, save cost and keep document integrity.

Secure Personal Information: Blockchain technology provide more security to personal information like aadhar no, DOB, etc. other identifying document which need to more security. It is free from lost, hacking, tampering chances happen in traditional system. It will very helpful in education, travelling, finance, healthcare system (Devi Parameswari et al., 2021).

Voting System: Traditional voting system has lot of demerit like one person can vote two times but using public ledger system it is guarantee that one person can't vote two times. Only applicable voters are vote and vote can't be tempered. It will make system more user suitable and user can click one button in his/her smartphone to vote. It will create system more transparent and reduced the election cost.

Government Benefits: Government use blockchain to verify some financial transaction, identify user identity for welfare scheme, social security, and public distribution system to monitor or track the beneficiaries by the administration of government benefits. It will enhance the system to reduce fraud and user get directly benefited through digital transaction (Hou et al., 2017).

Medical: Using blockchain doctor and medical professional can easy access the medical record anywhere any time it is helpful to treatment the patient anywhere. It will help the system to speed up the medical procedure. It is also helpful in if patient have an insurance covariance then hospitals check the validity and get treat directly there is no physical verification needed (Ben Fekih et al., 2020).

Artist Royalties: Blockchain technology provide tracking facility like music and film files distributed on the internet sure that artist are paid for music work. It will also create transparency to the system nowhere same file can exists leads to reduced piracy.

Supply Chain System: Blockchain provide major role in supply chain system to keep monitoring Product, tampering, delay, etc. everyone in the system can track the product at any point of time. So using smart contract concept in blockchain make supply chain more autonomous (Pournader et al., 2020).

Internet of Things (IoT): IoT collect data from different place and store in centralized place. IoT device are less computational power and connected over network. Blockchain provide security to IoT data which more secure. With the help of IoT device in blockchain we can make automatic smart agriculture system, smart drug monitoring system (Cho et al., 2019).

Date Storage: Instead of centralized system blockchain provide decentralized way to data storage to provide higher security and integrity of data. Due to decentralized, it will be difficult to hack and wipe out all the data through network. The storage cost also reduced through blockchain (Chaudhary et al., 2021).

Consensus Technique in Blockchain

It's a mechanism called decision making for group, in which individual of group create and agreed the decision that works best for the rest of them. It is a kind of rule where individuals need to support the majority decision, whether they liked it or not. Consensus mechanism do not agree with majority node, but it agree to one that provide benefit all of the node connected to network, that's why network always wining. The problem arise with byzantine is to reach an agreement. When a single node found to fault occur then node cannot come to agreement or higher difficulty value. This type of problem never found in consensus mechanism therefore consensus protocol have biggest advantage to support fault tolerance. Different consensus mechanism describe as.

PoW: PoW stand for proof of work. Whenever a user create a transaction the "miners" like supercomputer is trying to solve a difficult problem in term of Puzzle to verify it. When a node is solve the problem and doing hard work to mining a single block get reward some value of coin. The concept behind to miner get lesser coin over time, it ensure that such smaller incentives to create less chance of the 51% attack. The majority bond of the miners of PoW is highly strong that's why the possibility of the community is more centralized. When all minor will solve the puzzle after that new block is created and confirm transaction therefore add these new block to blockchain. There are some popular cryptocurrency used Proof-of-work is Bitcoin here it take 10 minutes to create a new block, Litecoin, Ethereum used very less. PoW provides DDoS security and lowers the overall stake mining (Gervais et al., 2016).

PoS: PoS stand for proof-of-stack. A user is stimulate to spend more whereas until he become a validator to create new block. The actual mining capability depend on single node based on he has already has how many coin. The 51% attack is grotesquely smashing in proof-of-stack method and the majority stake holders of PoS is not strong that's why PoS community is more decentralized. In PoW the mining process get higher computational power result leads to high energy consumption so using PoS eliminate the drawback of the PoW. Here all block get validated before network append other block to blockchain ledger. The interesting thing is to miners can joining mining process using own available coin to stake. So in PoS all individual node can mine or validate new block on the basis of own available coin possession. In this process there is chance that if you have more coin then your mining chance is greater. This process happen entirely randomly. Not every minor can participate in the staking. If you have reserve some amount of coin in your wallet then you were qualified the condition of node on the network. Onward there is voting system for choosing the validators. The ratio of mining block to coin is if you have already 15% coin then there is possibility that you can mine 15% new block. This technique doesn't need to heavy hardware backup. It also decrees the threat of a 51% attack. PoS is using by many cryptocurrency like PIVX, NavCoin, Straits (Gaži et al., 2019).

PBFT: Practical Byzantine Fault Tolerance working based on state machine. This algorithm assume that from starting there could be possible failure in the network and at least some individual node can malfunction at certain time. However every node in the system arrange in specific order. Pickup one node as primary and other one is backup. Every information found in network are verify therefore communication level is very high. Using this process the system can reach if one node getting compromised then every node reach an agreement through majority voting.

SBFT: Simplified Byzantine Fault Tolerance works on block will take every transaction, batch them same as another block then validate all of them together. To validate all transactions, the generator implements certain rule that are followed by all nodes. A block verifier validate them and append their own signature to them. As a result, any block that is missing any one of the keys will be rejected (Bach et al., 2018).

Attack Possible on Blockchain

In 2019, the white hat hacker found 43 bugs in different blockchain and cryptocurrency just in 25 days. They also found some vulnerabilities in platform such as Coinbase, EOS, and Tezos (Hasanova et al., 2019).

DDoS Attack: It is hard to execute but possible when attacking, hacker sending thousands of request at a time to bring down the server and aiming to break the network mining pools, e-wallet, crypto exchange and other financial services. Using DDoS botnets blockchain also hack in its application layer. In 2017 found that Bitfinex suffered from huge DDoS attack. It has been caught by IOTA foundation which is launch the token on the platform when Bitfinex announce the attack.

Transaction Malleability Attacks: This attack came in picture when victim paying twice. Every transaction in a bitcoin network has hash that is transaction ID. If hacker change the transaction ID, they can send the transaction with modified hash to network and have it confirmed ago the original transaction. If transaction is successful then sender think about initial transaction has failed whereas fund still cut form sender account thereafter sender send the money again which is because same amount deduction twice. This hack is successful where two transaction are grant by minors. This problem is solved by bitcoin by introducing segregated witness process.

Routing Attacks: It will have impact on both nodes as well as whole network. The idea behind of hack is to tamper transaction before them to peers. It is very difficult to other node to detect tampering and hacker portioned the network which is unable connect each other.

Sybil Attacks: It is a kind of attack where many identifiers have assign to same node. The network has trust less and all request is send to a number of nodes. When attack happen then attacker take control of network. The victim node get surrounded by fake node that cause problem and capture the transaction. It is very difficult to find attack and prevent from it.

Eclipse Attacks: This kind of attack contain large number of IP addresses or have a distributed botnet. Then the hacker try to overwrite the address in the tried table of the user and wait till restarted. After restarting all ongoing connection of user node can diverted to the IP address controlled under hacker.

Role of IoT in Healthcare System

The internet of things (IoT) is a collection of linked computing devices, such as electronic and mechanical equipment, objects, living things, and people that allow data transmission over a network without requiring people-to-people or people-to-computer interaction. Internet of Things infrastructure make up from Internet based smart devices that rely on embedded systems, which include microprocessor, sensors, and communication tools, to gather, send, and act on the data they receive from their surroundings. It allow allows IoT devices to exchange their acquired sensor data from connecting to IoT gateway, which either sends the gathered sensor data to the cloud for analysis or performs local analysis (Kodali et al., 2015). These gadgets occasionally interact with other similar device and take action based on the data they exchange. Before the Internet of Things, patients could only communicate with doctors face-to-face, over the phone, or by text. There was no feasible mechanism for medical professionals or facilities to continuously evaluate patient health and offer advice. Recent COVID-19 scenario it is very challenging task to treat patient physically therefore using IoT device we have provide solution of these challenging task with the help of blockchain based supplychain to sharing information between all participating entity (Sabukunze et al., 2021).

IoT for Patient: With the use of smart wearable like pedometers and other wirelessly connected medical equipment like cardiovascular and blood pressure rate monitor, cuffs, glucometers, oxymeter, thermometer, etc., patients can receive individualised care. These devices can be set up to remind users to monitor changes in their blood pressure, appointments, and a variety of other things. IoT has changed people's life by making it feasible to regularly follow medical conditions, especially those of older patients. This has a big influence on single-person households and families. When someone's routine is interrupted or altered, their alarm function notifies worried family members and medical staff.

IoT for Doctors: By deploying wearable's and other IoT-enabled home monitoring devices, doctors may more effectively keep an eye on their patients' health. They can keep an eye on a patient's compliance with their treatment plan or any immediate medical requirements. Thanks to IoT, medical staff may now actively interact with patients and be more watchful. IoT device data can help clinicians select the most suitable therapeutic approach for patients and achieve desired outcomes.

IoT for Hospitals: There are numerous other applications for IoT devices in hospitals besides patient health monitoring. The real-time position of medical equipment like wheelchairs, defibrillators, nebulizers, oxygen pumps, and other monitoring equipment is tracked using IoT devices tagged with sensors. Real-time analysis can also be done of the placement of medical personnel at various sites. Patients in hospitals are extremely concerned about the spread of infections. Patient infection can be avoided with the aid of IoT-enabled hygiene monitoring equipment. IoT devices are also useful for asset management tasks like controlling pharmacy inventory and checking refrigerator temperatures as well as controlling humidity and temperature in the environment.

IoT for Insurance Companies: With IoT-connected intelligent devices, health insurers have a lot of options. Health monitoring device data can be used by insurance companies' underwriting and claims departments. They will be able to identify candidates for underwriting and discover fraud claims thanks to this data. IoT devices improve communication between insurance organizations and their clients by increasing transparency in the policy, billing, claim settlement, and risk evaluation processes. In virtue of IoT-captured data-driven actions in all functional procedures, customers will have enough transparency into the underlying justification for every decision made and the outcomes of the process. Customers of insurance firms might be compensated for utilizing and sharing patient records generated by IoT devices.

Customers can receive benefits for using IoT devices to track their normal activities, adherence to treatment plans, and general health measures. This will drastically lower claims for insurance. Insurance firms may be able to verify claims using IoT devices and the data they collect. Therefore IoT has various advantage in healthcare field like cost reduction, improved treatment facility and make healthcare system more reliable (Kashani et al., 2021).

SMART CONTRACT FOR SMART HEALTHCARE SYSTEM

Smart contract is the heart of blockchain. In 2015 Ethereum blockchain came in picture with smart contract feature get more popular. Smart contract first time invented in 1990 by Nick Szabo. Smart contract resolve the concept of mining in bitcoin. Basically smart contract is the contract between two party without involvement of third party is nothing but a piece of code or script written in high level programming language called solidity programming language that run on Ethereum like c, c++, java, and python. Solidity was introduced in 2014 by Gavin wood. It is also called statically typed curly braces programming. Statically means it support inheritance, libraries and complex user defined type. Using solidity we can develop smart contract like pet adaptation system, voting system, financial transaction, crowd funding, blind auction, supply chain, etc. (Wang et al., 2019).

It work on the basis of deterministic machine model if condition satisfy then it will automatically executed and certain outcome came without any third party involvement or time loss and it will move from one state to other state. The working script like "if/when…then..." written inside blockchain. Computer network execute action based on satisfying condition and verify. Then the blockchain is update the transaction when transaction completed successfully. No one can the transaction and only permitted node can view the result. Example a doctor treat patient remotely and monitoring patient health status using IoT in Figure 6. A contract between patient, hospital and Insurance Company. When patient needed treatment then approach to hospital and doctor view the current health status of patient and according to treat them. If needed more treatment then doctor fit the IoT sensing device at patient body therefore device keep capture the data and process them and send to ledger of blockchain therefore smart contract update the information and doctor can easily view the health status of patient remotely. If patient already take a health insurance then hospital directly collect the money from insurance company because of whole process are in the form of supply chain and enable to view transaction status any point of time by participating authority. There are many benefits of smart contract like it will provide the system to speed up, more efficient, and high accuracy because once a condition is satisfy then action automatically executed immediate whereas contract in digital form there is no time spent on rectifying errors that find in manually filling in document. One more benefit is trust and transparency because there is no third party involve in between transaction and transaction is share in encrypted format. One more benefit in term of security because of record are store in block with cryptographic link chain so if hacker want to hack or modify single data means entire chain alter for single character and smart contract save the time and cost because everything is automatic.

KEY MANAGEMENT USING SMART CONTRACT TO UPGRADE THE SYSTEM SECURITY

Healthcare system is a common platform to provide treatment facility in which many level of entity involve to ensure the better functioning of the system. Assume

Figure 6. Smart contract for healthcare system

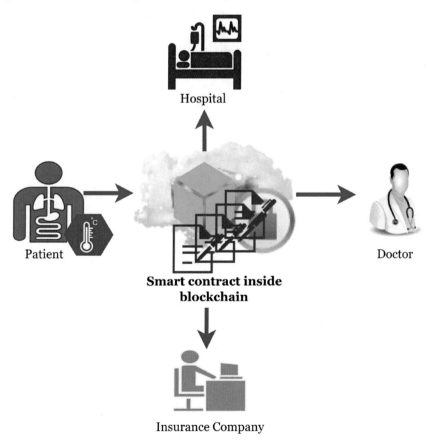

a new hospital (H_N) want to join the system however in traditional healthcare system there is lack of proper authentication scheme therefore sharing information between participating entities at risk and possibility of security breach. Here we have discus a key management based security protocol to ensure the security of system. When new hospital (H_N) want to join the system then H_N first request to certificate authority (CA) to grant certificate whereas after receiving request first of all certificate authority verify the H_N secret parameter after that CA check the public key of new entity (PUH_N) along with its identity (IDH_N) already exist in authority database or not. It will confirm that new entity already not be the part of the system therefore CA issue the certificate of requesting entity H_N as ($CERTH_N$). The certificate consist of various parameter like name of new entity (H_N), public key of new entity (PUH_N), identity of new entity (IDH_N), date of certification validation, version number, name of certificate authority, and digital signature of CA. When new entity once receive the certificate then it will publically send to leader validator node (L_V) node for verification of certificate to ensure certificate is issue by certificate authority or not (Using validator selection algorithm (VSA) chose L_V publically). If verification is successful then L_V ensure that public key of new entity PUH_N along with H_N is true, then L_V insert the public key (PUH_N) of new entity on behalf of identity of (IDH_N) in the ledger and update the smart contract thereafter remaining participating entity get touch with L_V to fetch the most recent updated copy of smart contract. Figure 7 given key management based updated scheme and ensure security of system in term of only authorized entity be the part of existing chain of blockchain.

Figure 7. Key management using smart contract

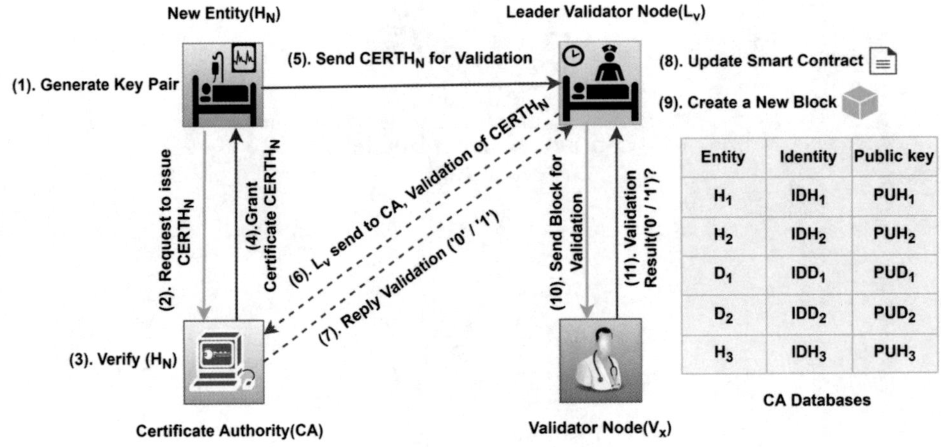

CONCLUSION

Healthcare system is the essential platform to provide better treatment facility to the patient therefore need to redevelop time to time and make smart healthcare system using latest technology. Using blockchain with IoT feature to rebuild the system automatic, accurate, efficient and easy for diagnosis. There are many level of monitoring body involve in proper functioning of these system however information sharing between participating entity without verifying is at risk even fraud happen, and sometimes attack happen on IoT process data even blockchain also hence security aspect is one of major challenging task in healthcare system. In this paper we have proposed an idea about key management technique to ensure security of the system from unauthorized access so that information sharing between only participating entity are secure, role of blockchain technology and IoT device for easy and proper treatment. The future scope of this scheme is implement in ruler area and provide the advice and treatment by big city to village.

REFERENCES

Bach, L. M., Mihaljevic, B., & Zagar, M. (2018, May). Comparative analysis of blockchain consensus algorithms. In *2018 41st International Convention on Information and Communication Technology, Electronics and Microelectronics (MIPRO)* (pp. 1545-1550). IEEE. 10.23919/MIPRO.2018.8400278

Ben Fekih, R., & Lahami, M. (2020, June). Application of blockchain technology in healthcare: a comprehensive study. In *International Conference on Smart Homes and Health Telematics* (pp. 268-276). Springer. 10.1007/978-3-030-51517-1_23

Berentsen, A. (2019). *Aleksander berentsen recommends "bitcoin: a peer-to-peer electronic cash system" by Satoshi Nakamoto. In 21st Century Economics*. Springer.

Budida, D. A. M., & Mangrulkar, R. S. (2017, March). Design and implementation of smart HealthCare system using IoT. In *2017 International Conference on Innovations in Information, Embedded and Communication Systems (ICIIECS)* (pp. 1-7). IEEE. 10.1109/ICIIECS.2017.8275903

Chamola, V., Hassija, V., Gupta, V., & Guizani, M. (2020). A comprehensive review of the COVID-19 pandemic and the role of IoT, drones, AI, blockchain, and 5G in managing its impact. *IEEE Access : Practical Innovations, Open Solutions*, 8, 90225–90265. doi:10.1109/ACCESS.2020.2992341

Chaudhary, B., & Singh, K. (2021). A Blockchain enabled location-privacy preserving scheme for vehicular ad-hoc networks. *Peer-to-Peer Networking and Applications*, *14*(5), 3198–3212. doi:10.100712083-021-01079-5

Cho, S., & Lee, S. (2019, January). Survey on the Application of BlockChain to IoT. In *2019 International Conference on Electronics, Information, and Communication (ICEIC)* (pp. 1-2). IEEE. 10.23919/ELINFOCOM.2019.8706369

De Aguiar, E. J., Faiçal, B. S., Krishnamachari, B., & Ueyama, J. (2020). A survey of blockchain-based strategies for healthcare. *ACM Computing Surveys*, *53*(2), 1–27. doi:10.1145/3376915

Devi Parameswari, C., & Mandadi, V. (2021). Public distribution system based on blockchain using solidity. In *Innovative Data Communication Technologies and Application* (pp. 175–183). Springer. doi:10.1007/978-981-15-9651-3_15

Dhakal, S., Jaafar, F., & Zavarsky, P. (2019, January). Private blockchain network for IoT device firmware integrity verification and update. In *2019 IEEE 19th International Symposium on High Assurance Systems Engineering (HASE)* (pp. 164-170). IEEE. 10.1109/HASE.2019.00033

Dwivedi, S. K., Amin, R., & Vollala, S. (2020). Blockchain based secured information sharing protocol in supply chain management system with key distribution mechanism. *Journal of Information Security and Applications*, *54*, 102554. doi:10.1016/j.jisa.2020.102554

Dwivedi, S. K., Roy, P., Karda, C., Agrawal, S., & Amin, R. (2021). Blockchain-based internet of things and industrial IoT: A comprehensive survey. *Security and Communication Networks*, *2021*, 2021. doi:10.1155/2021/7142048

Gaži, P., Kiayias, A., & Zindros, D. (2019, May). Proof-of-stake sidechains. In *2019 IEEE Symposium on Security and Privacy (SP)* (pp. 139-156). IEEE. 10.1109/SP.2019.00040

Gervais, A., Karame, G. O., Wüst, K., Glykantzis, V., Ritzdorf, H., & Capkun, S. (2016, October). On the security and performance of proof of work blockchains. In *Proceedings of the 2016 ACM SIGSAC conference on computer and communications security* (pp. 3-16). 10.1145/2976749.2978341

Hasanova, H., Baek, U. J., Shin, M. G., Cho, K., & Kim, M. S. (2019). A survey on blockchain cybersecurity vulnerabilities and possible countermeasures. *International Journal of Network Management*, *29*(2), e2060. doi:10.1002/nem.2060

Hou, H. (2017, July). The application of blockchain technology in E-government in China. In *2017 26th International Conference on Computer Communication and Networks (ICCCN)* (pp. 1-4). IEEE. 10.1109/ICCCN.2017.8038519

Kashani, M. H., Madanipour, M., Nikravan, M., Asghari, P., & Mahdipour, E. (2021). A systematic review of IoT in healthcare: Applications, techniques, and trends. *Journal of Network and Computer Applications*, *192*, 103164. doi:10.1016/j.jnca.2021.103164

Khan, A. G., Zahid, A. H., Hussain, M., Farooq, M., Riaz, U., & Alam, T. M. (2019, November). A journey of WEB and Blockchain towards the Industry 4.0: An Overview. In *2019 International Conference on Innovative Computing (ICIC)* (pp. 1-7). IEEE. 10.1109/ICIC48496.2019.8966700

Kodali, R. K., Swamy, G., & Lakshmi, B. (2015, December). An implementation of IoT for healthcare. In 2015 IEEE Recent Advances in Intelligent Computational Systems (RAICS) (pp. 411-416). IEEE. doi:10.1109/RAICS.2015.7488451

Kouhizadeh, M., & Sarkis, J. (2018). Blockchain practices, potentials, and perspectives in greening supply chains. *Sustainability (Basel)*, *10*(10), 3652. doi:10.3390u10103652

Liu, M., Wu, K., & Xu, J. J. (2019). How will blockchain technology impact auditing and accounting: Permissionless versus permissioned blockchain. *Current Issues in Auditing*, *13*(2), A19–A29. doi:10.2308/ciia-52540

Lockl, J., Schlatt, V., Schweizer, A., Urbach, N., & Harth, N. (2020). Toward trust in Internet of Things ecosystems: Design principles for blockchain-based IoT applications. *IEEE Transactions on Engineering Management*, *67*(4), 1256–1270. doi:10.1109/TEM.2020.2978014

Madaan, L., Kumar, A., & Bhushan, B. (2020, April). Working principle, application areas and challenges for blockchain technology. In *2020 IEEE 9th international conference on communication systems and network technologies (CSNT)* (pp. 254-259). IEEE. 10.1109/CSNT48778.2020.9115794

Meng, T., Zhao, Y., Wolter, K., & Xu, C. Z. (2021). On consortium blockchain consistency: A queueing network model approach. *IEEE Transactions on Parallel and Distributed Systems*, *32*(6), 1369–1382. doi:10.1109/TPDS.2021.3049915

Norman, M. D., Karavas, Y. G., & Reed, H. (2018, July). The emergence of trust and value in public blockchain networks. In *IX International Conference on Complex Systems* (p. 22). Academic Press.

Peng, L., Feng, W., Yan, Z., Li, Y., Zhou, X., & Shimizu, S. (2021). Privacy preservation in permissionless blockchain: A survey. *Digital Communications and Networks*, *7*(3), 295–307. doi:10.1016/j.dcan.2020.05.008

Pournader, M., Shi, Y., Seuring, S., & Koh, S. L. (2020). Blockchain applications in supply chains, transport and logistics: A systematic review of the literature. *International Journal of Production Research*, *58*(7), 2063–2081. doi:10.1080/00 207543.2019.1650976

Sabukunze, I. D., Setyohadi, D. B., & Sulistyoningsih, M. (2021, April). Designing an IoT based smart monitoring and emergency alert system for COVID19 patients. In *2021 6th International Conference for Convergence in Technology (I2CT)* (pp. 1-5). IEEE. 10.1109/I2CT51068.2021.9418078

Tosh, D. K., Shetty, S., Liang, X., Kamhoua, C. A., Kwiat, K. A., & Njilla, L. (2017, May). Security implications of blockchain cloud with analysis of block withholding attack. In *2017 17th IEEE/ACM International Symposium on Cluster, Cloud and Grid Computing (CCGRID)* (pp. 458-467). IEEE. 10.1109/CCGRID.2017.111

Wang, S., Ouyang, L., Yuan, Y., Ni, X., Han, X., & Wang, F. Y. (2019). Blockchain-enabled smart contracts: Architecture, applications, and future trends. *IEEE Transactions on Systems, Man, and Cybernetics. Systems*, *49*(11), 2266–2277. doi:10.1109/TSMC.2019.2895123

Wüst, K., & Gervais, A. (2018, June). Do you need a blockchain? In *2018 Crypto Valley Conference on Blockchain Technology (CVCBT)* (pp. 45-54). IEEE. 10.1109/ CVCBT.2018.00011

Zhu, S., Cai, Z., Hu, H., Li, Y., & Li, W. (2019). zkCrowd: A hybrid blockchain-based crowdsourcing platform. *IEEE Transactions on Industrial Informatics*, *16*(6), 4196–4205. doi:10.1109/TII.2019.2941735

Zou, Y., Meng, T., Zhang, P., Zhang, W., & Li, H. (2020). Focus on blockchain: A comprehensive survey on academic and application. *IEEE Access : Practical Innovations, Open Solutions*, *8*, 187182–187201. doi:10.1109/ACCESS.2020.3030491

Chapter 4
Significance of Cyber Security in Healthcare Systems

Anuj Singh

ⓘ https://orcid.org/0000-0001-8880-780X
Graphic Era University (Deemed), India

Somjit Mandal
National Chiao Tung University, Hsinchu, Taiwan

Kamlesh Chandra Purohit
Graphic Era University (Deemed), India

ABSTRACT

The healthcare sector is one of the industries most vulnerable to cyberattacks. healthcare cybercrime is significantly expanding as it relates to healthcare services that are digitally enabled, and it aims to exploit security flaws and vulnerabilities. Technology improvements have exposed the healthcare sector to a wide range of extremely dangerous threats, such as ransomware. Ransomware, a sort of hack that targets both organisations and individual people, has become more prevalent recently as a result of its effective results. There has been a significant improvement in its disputes over the previous several years. The study includes answers as well as a complete overview of ransomware attacks. The main goal of this study is to classify the cyberattack defences employed by healthcare programmes to stop ransomware, such as blockchain and machine learning. Studies investigating information security, medical organisations, and security firms will all benefit scientifically from the study.

INTRODUCTION

Healthcare is an extremely specialised profession that handles a lot of sensitive personal data. In our internet-driven age where everything is handled over the internet,

DOI: 10.4018/978-1-6684-6646-9.ch004

this information is even more crucial (Thamer & Alubady, 2021). Healthcare firms confront issues dealing with very sensitive information. They continually fight rising cyber hazards and adjust to the digital transition while adhering to tighter laws. The healthcare industry is currently quite dynamic. hospitals are joining networks, forming alliances, and undergoing an extraordinary degree of merger acquisition consolidation. This is an exciting time in healthcare because healthcare is changing new technologies are being developed daily that allow patients to track their own health patients are demanding more individualised care, and health information exchanges are being implemented. It's really not a question of if a breach occurs but rather where now that we all know that health care institutions are very vulnerable. Now that healthcare is complicated, personal health records are being prescribed online health communities, and it's getting worse, sensitive and personal information is being shared with a variety of technologies, and every time it's shared, there's a cyber risk involved, so healthcare organisations need to have measures in place to stop hackers from gaining access to that sensitive information (Maurya et al., 2018). Hospitals are targets of cyberattacks, which are on the rise. The abundance of sensitive data makes it a gold mine for cybercriminals. First off, the health care sector is ripe for hacking since patient records can be purchased on the dark web for up to $1,000 Medical records contain a range of A patient's medical data being stolen or compromised might have long-lasting effects. birth dates, credit card information, social security numbers, residences, and email addresses. Malicious software, sometimes known as malware, is merely software designed with the goal to harm systems, steal data, or generally cause chaos. Malware has infected more than 88% of the healthcare industries as a whole. 88%, now that's a lot. 96% of ransomware attacks on healthcare organisations target medical treatment centres because they are easy targets (Thamer et al., 2021). Healthcare had the fifth-highest number of ransomware assaults out of the 18 industries surveyed, and it completely destroys the healthcare institution.

The healthcare institution where it occurs presently according to article more than half of the healthcare industry and has a network security grade of less than a C-GRADE (Venter et al., 2019). This indicates that when they were evaluated, the security scores they received reflected whether or not the company could protect its data from data breaches, and obviously healthcare has not made that a priority. The healthcare industry ranks 15th and is vulnerable to social engineering techniques. Healthcare workers tend to be very trusting, but social engineering is really the ability to persuade someone to give you their personal or private information by using dishonest tactics (Zakus et al., 2014). Simple tasks like timely updating security patches were a problem in 63% of the healthcare entities surveyed. This is just one of the basic things that health care institutions need to do when anyone needs to do to ensure that they're guarding against whatever the latent threat is. fashion possible schedule it make sure somebody's doing it unfortunately in healthcare there's some When a disaster strikes in the United States or any other country, hackers ramp up their activities because they believe that people won't be aware of what's happening. In January 2020, there was a breach at LabCorp involving 10,000 company documents that were stolen. This is typically not done because there are other pressing issues. However, in this time of coronavirus, and some panicking things going on in the case of coronavirus (Yamany et al., 2022). hacker are doing what's calling called password spraying campaigns as part of their cyber operations and what password spraying is it's basically a simple tactic that's called a brute-force attack (Gautam & Jain, 2015) when the hacker attempts to get access to the organization's systems by testing a small number of frequently used passwords on a big number of accounts The hacker assumes that among a big group of people, there is likely to be at least one common password that many of these people share (He et al., 2021). That is an excellent reason why organisations should educate their staff on how to create unique and strong passwords. some figures, which are rather frightening In the previous three years, 93% of health care organisations have had a data breach, and 57% have experienced more than five breaches.

HEALTHCARE SYSTEMS

now health care offers many opportunities for hackers it does because there are a lot of different entry points for hackers to gain access of a system network is one of good as the weakest link and in healthcare and hacker (Donnan, 2019) know that all devices use IP as a part of network These gadgets might be risky, for instance in a conventional operating room all of these digital devices are used and a lot of these different things have an IP address and any device with an IP address is potentially a device that can cyber criminal hack and anything from patient monitoring devices to x-ray tech to the timing devices whether it be a clock to the oxygen that's going to a patient and the scary part is that the researchers found that there were close to 50,000 malicious events and 723 malicious sort sorry Melissa malicious source IP addresses that were able to compromise devices and (Usak et al., 2020) all that means is if a hacker can get access to the IP address on a device they have entry into the hospital's network in most cases or at bare minimum into wreaking havoc with that one device and the compromised devices that were found were anything from radiology to software image to imaging software to firewalls to web cameras to mail servers but you can use your imagination because everything in medicine just about everything these days has an IP address now there is a wonderful Institute called the (Cimpanu, 2020) Ponemon Institute the conducts independent research on data protection and they do it for the healthcare industry as well and what they did most recently was a global study of 350 healthcare companies in 11 countries and these are some of the things that they found they asked the question if your organization had suffered a data breach that involved the loss or theft of patient data within the (Cipanu, 2020) last 24 months and if you look at this 91% people 990 people 91 percent of these health care institutions said that they did suffer a breach within the past 24 months and 40% of them said that they had actually suffered more than five breaches which is astounding they asked also how was this patient data successfully targeted and what they found out was that all (He et al., 2021) departments within a healthcare institution are vulnerable it doesn't matter if you're in building and billing an insurance it doesn't matter if you're in scheduling it doesn't matter if you're fulfilling prescriptions none of the departments seems to be immune to the hackers the next thing that they wanted to know is that when you had a breach how did it happen and if you look at this very carefully what you're going to see is that lost and stolen devices had were contributed to the breach 96% of the time and spear-phishing 88% of the time and the things that is unique about these two items is they all info they all involve employees and employees seem to be the weakest link here for the majority of the data breaches spyware accounted for 29% zero day attacks which no one can know healthcare care institution really can stop accounted for 29% and all of these other things were really not associated with employees so the health care institutions what security threats worry them the most employee negligence was the answer in 70% of the time and in fact employees are responsible for about 51% of the breaches and on purpose obviously but 51% of the breaches that's a lot and in most cases it's unintentional it's an employee doing something that (Cipanu, 2020) normally do not really thinking about it not being aware of their surroundings or who's watching them put the passwords in unintentional employee action and that also involves stolen items now the average price tag for dealing with an individual breach ranges from about 10,000 to more than a million.

Healthcare institutions surveyed had (Georgiadou et al., 2021) that they experienced five or more breaches in a 24 month period that's an awful lot of money now the cost of this insecurity the high cost of not having cybersecurity mitigation in place is has a lot of different factors first there's the cost of outside security consulting if you consult (He et al., 2021) with a firm that can be around two hundred and fifty thousand dollars and the cost of reporting the data breach to the state and federal authorities is around four dollars per patient there's a cost of cleaning up the mess a cost of daily disruption there's a (He et al., 2021) cost of ID theft monitoring that runs around ten dollars a patient usually there's a class action lawsuit associated with it and the e-discovery phase just that phase is between 250 and 500 thousand dollars and if you lose the lawsuit the cost can be astronomical also individual states will add to the financial world because the individual (Hedayati, 2012) states have different investigation fees and different fines so you want to make sure that you have a good cybersecurity plan in place now the cost of being secure is relatively low educating employees is probably going to be your largest expense if you want and you what you should do is be encrypting all of your devices so that the breach that happened at Dartmouth did didn't really it wouldn't really happen if your devices are encrypted (Foley et al., 2003) then the hackers have a much more difficult time getting their data and the average cost of an encryption of a single device is around 150 dollars which means that the cost of enterprise encryption for the whole healthcare institution runs usually between (San Diego, 2007) 250 and 500 thousand dollars remember the average writer has at least five breaches which can mount to millions of dollars so this seemed to be seems to be a cost-effective way to ensure that you don't have problems now this is a perspective over the last 12 months and the things that about education of employees we need to educate people coming up and the ranks that will provide cybersecurity to us (Maher, 2011) education is definitely the best bang for your buck if you can prevent 51% of these breaches just by educating your employee you're going to do a lot in terms of keeping your health care institution safe now .cyber criminals are pretty devious but they recognize two (Schmitz, 2018) critical factors the first is that health care institutions manage a treasure trove of financially lucrative personal information and before each patient record can go for as high as $1,000 a record on the dark web the second thing is that health care institutions don't have the resources or the technology or the processes in place to prevent and detect attacks remember the average time of detecting attack was about 236 days they can't protect their patient data adequately so what do we need to do well the first is to establish a security culture because ongoing cybersecurity training and (Angst & Block, 2017) NGH education emphasize that every member of the team is important and every member of the team is responsible for knowing what to do and what not to do to keep their records safe the second is to protect mobile devices because an increasing number of health care providers are using mobile devices at work an encryption and other protective measures are critical to ensure that any information on these devices is secure (Oso et al., 2019) the third is to maintain good computer habits make sure that new employees who are on boarding should be trained on the best practices for their computer used including installing software and operating system maintenance number four is to use a firewall anything that is connected to the Internet should have an active firewall in place now number five is install and maintain antivirus software simply installing software is it's not enough you need to continuously update the software to (Dempster & Eaton-Lee, 2006) make sure that you are getting the best possible protection at any given point in time so (Karapapas et al., 2020) when those popups occurs make sure that you either alert the IT team number six is planned for the unexpected you know you never know what these hackers are going to do you never know if your date is going to be stolen so if you back up your systems regularly restore from your backup files in a (Le et al., 2018) very short period of time now most organizations consider should consider storing backup information away from the main system if at all possible because you want to make sure that you always have a place that you can go to get your data back now number seven is to control access to protected health information what happens is normally it's the (Kumar et al., 2019) IT people who grant access to those who need to view or use the data but the problem is when employ change jobs or an employee is no longer with the institution they forget to change those privileges so make sure that control access to whoever can control the access to whoever has access to protected information and only let them see what they absolutely 'need to see now it is important to (Akarca et al., 2019) used strong passwords and change them regularly remember of password spraying you don't want to have a password that is like anybody else's and have a password that is difficult to (Akcora et al., 2019) guess that is easy to remember and that is fairly complex and includes symbols capital letters numbers limit network access any software applications or other additions to the existing system should not be installed by company staff member without prior consent from the proper organizational authorities don't let anyone to use system who doesn't have the authority to install software and finally small number on authorized is to control the physical access data can be breached (Jabbar, 2021) when any sort of physical device is stolen and computer and other electronics that contain protected information should be kept in locked rooms in secured areas and don't forget your trash the trash is a treasure trove of personal information make sure that you shred it make sure that never put personal patient information in the trash and just generally be careful of your physical surroundings (Thamer & Alubady, 2021). Health care institutions need to have cyber security and healthcare informatics specialists on board to do this they need to have people who are educated who understand (Thamer & Alubady, 2021) healthcare who understand the nuances of the healthcare system and they understand computer technology and cyber security and they know how to protect those systems and this is why you know all the (Thamer & Alubady, 2021) HIPAA basics but keeping your medical practice compliant with hey're requirements and complicated legal statutes seems (Almashhadani et al., 2019) next to impossible it's so confusing and frustrating it's no wonder most practices would rather just bury their head in the sand and until now they've gotten away with it since there's been practically no enforcement of HIPAA regulations but those days are over the Department of Health and (Hirano & Kobayashi, 2019) Human Services Office for Civil Rights recently hired consultants to audit the HIPAA privacy and security compliance of medical practices all over the country and that's just the tip of the iceberg between audits like these and state level enforcement efforts breaches of protected health information are being discovered every day often resulting in large fines and class-action lawsuits the average cost of one of those large breaches in 2011 was 1.5 million dollars enough to bankrupt many practices not to mention the damages to their operations and reputations so you know you need to do something but how do you get compliant and where do you even start most IT companies know nothing about (Almashhadani et al., 2019) HIPAA compliance they'll just change everybody's passwords and tell you you're fine and hiring some consultant just to come in and point out all your problems is almost worse they won't be able to execute any of their solutions and will just leave you with some terrifying report that might just make you more liable for all the things you now know are (Hirano & Kobayashi, 2019) wrong what you need is someone who understands all the technical and legal nuances of HIPAA compliance inside and out who can actually implement all the right solutions to get and keep you HIPAA compliant in the most cost effective and sustainable way possible you need a professional you need someone who has been trained and someone who's understands HIPAA and understands healthcare institutions these are the (Akbanov et al., 2019) kind of things that these healthcare informatics and cyber security specialists study they look at emerging healthcare security threats they look at the security (Wani & Revathi, 2020) of medical devices they're trained in the state of incidence response they look at information sharing networks they look at mobile and digital care and what to do with those devices what are the challenges when using the cloud and what are the cyber security threats and challenges for the health insurance exchanges of which there many now (El Hajal et al., 2019) cybersecurity and healthcare informatics specialists do well they implement basic cybersecurity tools they fortify authentic authentication measures they used role-based administration you can read this as easily have very (Ghafir et al., 2018) specific skills that are associated with their very specialized education as well as they keep an eye on the future they're looking for the next big cybersecurity threat and helping you guard against it now cybersecurity and healthcare informatics personnel work together with healthcare providers and all of the associated businesses to be confident that every aspect of their operation is electronically secure

THE MOST REGULAR TYPES OF ATTACKS IN HEALTHCARE SYSTEMS

Phishing Attack: Phishing is a sort of cybersecurity assault in which hostile actors send messages while posing as a reliable person or organisation. Phishing communications trick users into installing harmful software, clicking on malicious links, or providing sensitive information such as login credentials (Sittig & Singh, 2016). The most popular sort of social engineering is phishing, which is a broad phrase that describes attempts to persuade or deceive computer users (Mujeye, 2022). Social engineering is a growing attack vector that is exploited in practically all security events. Phishing and other forms of social engineering are routinely combined with malware, code injection, and network attacks. A phishing attack begins with a message sent via email, social media, or another electronic communication channel (Mohammed et al., 2021). A phisher may specifically use social media to obtain background information on the victim's career and personal history. These sources are utilised to gather information on the potential victim, such as his or her name, occupation, email address, interests, and behaviours. Using this information, the phisher can create a credible phoney message. The victim regularly receives emails that appear to be from well-known persons or organisations. Infected attachments or links to unauthorised websites are used to initiate attacks. Attackers commonly create bogus websites that look to be operated by a legitimate organisation, such as the victim's employer.

Data in the healthcare industry is very valuable as a possible hacking target. Phishing is the process of using targeted communications (email/messaging) to exploit data for malevolent objectives. According to Arlington Research and Kaspersky, a number of research indicated that patients turned down telemedicine sessions owing to a lack of confidence in telehealth cybersecurity. This paper analyses peer-reviewed research (Mohurle & Patil, 2017) on phishing in the healthcare industry and presents findings from an internal assessment aimed at hospital workers. According to the poll, when using remote telemedicine, a third of physicians had the data on their patients compromised. In addition, 32% of respondents stated that cybersecurity issues and phishing attempts were brought on by third-party vendor weaknesses. There is mounting evidence that healthcare workers are particularly susceptible to phishing scams.

The majority of healthcare phishing attempts are reported to be carried out by email, while there have also been reports of assaults using social media and malicious advertising (Mohammed et al., 2021). These emails frequently look legitimate, and they direct employees to click on a link to a web page where they are prompted to

Figure 1. Ping attack

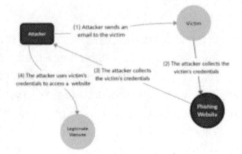

Figure 2. Types of phishing attack

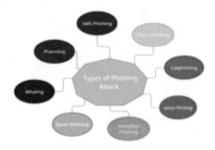

do anything that starts a virus download or enter their account and password. It's possible that virus downloads might not always contain ransomware. Keystroke loggers and adware are two kinds of surveillance software that can track passwords and usernames while keeping an eye on employees' internet behaviour (Runciman, 2020). By installing malicious software that opens doors for hackers, the network of an organisation can be accessed remotely. If phishing is used, the hacker is likely to obtain access to Protected Health Information (PHI) fairly immediately.

Ransomware Attack

Ransomware aims to block a user or organisation from accessing files on their computer. Ransomware is a category of malicious software that demands a ransom payment from the victim in exchange for not destroying or restricting access to (Akbanov et al., 2019) data or a computer system, typically by encrypting it. Usually, the ransom demand includes a timeframe. If the victim doesn't pay the ransom in a timely manner, the (Hirano & Kobayashi, 2019) data is permanently erased or the ransom price rises. Ransomware is employed in conjunction with a variety of programmes, including Crypto Locker and Crypt Wall. Locky, also known as Crypto Locker, is an exceptionally strong tool for encoding victims' sensitive data. This approach is being used by hackers to acquire a large number of cryptocurrencies. Most ransomware spreads via email attachments, although victims can possibly download any file from a compromised website (Wani & Revathi, 2020). When this malware is operating on a victim's computer, it locks it and encrypts its data files. When files are encrypted, a notification appears informing users how to obtain the decryption key in exchange for a ransom payment. Through a download from a spam email attachment, ransomware may access your network in one of the most frequent methods. The download then activates the ransomware virus, which then infects your machine. The use of social engineering techniques and installing (Mohurle & Patil, 2017) malicious software from the internet—either directly from a website or by clicking on deceptive advertising known as "malvertising"—are other methods of entrance. Chat messaging and detachable USB devices are two ways that malware may propagate. Even under normal operating conditions, criminal groups using ransomware pose a serious danger to the healthcare business, with potential implications including the interruption of key care facilities. Exfiltrating data before the ransomware is triggered, a tendency witnessed across all industries in 2020, poses an additional threat to victims. This risk is in addition to the chance of major important function interruption.

Types of Ransomware

In the (Hirano & Kobayashi, 2019) past, the two most frequent types of ransomware were crypto and locker. Extortion and ransomware as a service (RaaS) have recently gained in popularity among threat actors. In 2020, there will be four types of ransomware.

Locker ransomware: Computer systems are completely inaccessible due to locker ransomware. Utilizing stolen credentials and social engineering tactics, this version compromises systems. Threat actors prevent users from using the system until (Akbanov et al., 2019) they have acquired access and paid a ransom. "Online pages with inappropriate information were visited through your computer," stated a pop-up notice. Your computer can have a virus on it or it might be locked and cost money to open.

Crypto ransomware: crypto ransomware is more widespread and common than locker ransomware. It encrypts all or a portion of the computer's files and demands a ransom payment in exchange for the decryption key. Some more (El Hajal et al., 2019) recent variants infect networked, cloud, and shared storage as well. Crypto ransomware is distributed through a variety of ways, including phishing emails, rogue websites, and downloads

Double extortion ransomware: To force victims to pay a ransom, double extortion ransomware exports data while encrypting files (Ghafir et al., 2018). Attackers using double extortion ransomware threaten to reveal stolen data if their demands are not satisfied. This implies that the attacker retains control even if the victim is able to recover their data from a backup. Paying the ransom, however, does not ensure data protection because the attackers have access to the stolen data.

RaaS: Ransomware-as-a-Service refers to the practise (Mohurle & Patil, 2017) of criminals renting access to a ransomware variant from the ransomware's developer, who offers it as a paid service. Similar to the SaaS paradigm, RaaS producers publish their ransomware on deep dark web sites and then let people subscribe to it. The costs vary depending on the intricacy and power of the infection, but there is often a membership fee. An agreed-upon proportion of the ransom is delivered to the creator of the RaaS once members have infected computers and accumulated ransom payments. The RaaS (Ransomware-as-a-Service) business model allows attackers to rent out ransomware and the management infrastructure from malware developers. RaaS is a subset of MaaS, and the MaaS (Malware-as-a-Service) model is a risky extension of the SaaS (Software-as-a-Service) idea.

Table 1. traces the development of ransomware between 1989 and 2022, providing us to examine how new ransomware upgrades and variants appear every year.

HEALTHCARE VICTIMS BY RANSOMWARE

The healthcare industry emerged as a contentious target for BGH operators during the epidemic. A few foes, such as GRACEFUL SPIDER, TWISTED SPIDER, VIKING SPIDER, and TRAVELING SPIDER, have declared their aim to stay away from frontline healthcare organisations. Others, such as DOPPEL SPIDER, (Maniath et al., 2017) claimed that by disseminating decryption keys without charging a fee, any inadvertent attacks against a healthcare practitioner would be promptly eradicated. In September 2020, an event involving a hospital with roots in Germany led to such a reaction. In contrast of these claims, Crowd Strike Intelligence reported that 104 healthcare institutions were affected by 18 different BGH ransomware families in 2020, with TWISTED SPIDER utilising Maze and WIZARD SPIDER using Conti being the (Alhawi et al., 2018) most common. In certain instances, enemies may have eschewed attacking hospitals in favour of strikes against pharmaceutical and biomedical firms.

TWISTED SPIDER used its (Al-Haija et al., 2020) Maze and Egregor ransomware families to assault at least 26 healthcare victims, predominantly in the United States, as seen in Figure 3. WIZARD SPIDER used Ryuk and Conti to launch 25 assaults on the medical business. Despite a concentrated attempt by cybersecurity companies to disrupt Ryuk in September 2020, Ryuk was largely blamed for an excessive number of infections that targeted U.S.-based healthcare organisations throughout the month of October 2020. On October 28, 2020, the FBI issued a warning regarding attacks employing WIZARD SPIDER's TrickBot that might result in ransomware infections and disruptions to healthcare systems as a result of this spike.

PURPOSED HEALTHCARE SOLUTION FOR RANSOMWARE

Attacks on (Mohurle & Patil, 2017) health care facilities, services, and associated equipment pose one of the major threats to the health sector and put patient safety in peril. This chapter provides an overview of the research that offers technological

Table 1. Ransomware timeline from 1989 to 2020 (techtarget.com)

Year	Month	Ransomware Timeline (Name)
1989	DECEMBER	AIDS Trojan
2004	DECEMBER	GPCode
2006	MAY	Archievus
2011	SEPTEMBER	Win Lock
2012	AUGUST	Reveton
2013	SEPTEMBER	Crypto Locker
2014	APRIL	Crypto Wall
	MAY	CTB-Locker
	JUNE	Simple Locker
2015	FEBRUARY	Tesla Crypt
	SEPTEMBER	Locker Pin Chimera
	NOVEMBER	Linux.Encoder.1
2016	JANUARY	Ransom 32
	FEBRUARY	Locky
	MARCH	Petya SamSam
	ARPIL	Jigsaw
	JUNE	Zcryptor
	SEPTEMBER	Mamba
2017	JANUARY	Spora
	MAY	Jaff wannaCry
	JUNE	Goldeneya Notpetya
	OCTOBER	Bad Rabbit
2018	JANUARY	Gand Crab
	AUGUST	Ryuk
2019	ARPIL	REvil
	MAY	Maze RobbinHood
	DECEMBER	Tycoon
2020	AUGUST	DarkSide
	SEPTEMBER	Egregon

ransomware solutions to protect healthcare systems and lessen the impact of the assault. The next sections provide a range of answers to the various Ransomware assault types shown in Fig. 4, each of which has a distinct behaviour and a Ransomware countermeasure.

*Figure 3. Ransomware assaults in number of millions from 2016 to H1 2022
Source:www.statista.com)*

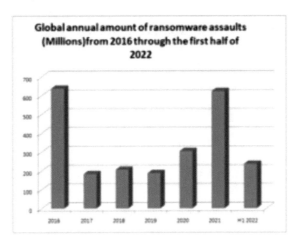

Blockchain: Previously Blockchain is usually utilised to perform a secure Blockchain exchange. In terms of healthcare applications, it improves patient security while enabling access to their medical records (Karapapas et al., 2020). Someone is more likely to target medical data transmitted in a hazardous environment. It is recommended that players in the health industry share information safely in order to facilitate information security. Because blockchain is eternal, it is more sophisticated than it appears. Because this technique's data structure provides an immutable reference for all confirmed state transitions, all information entering the network must be completely accurate and safe because it cannot be updated (Le & Wang, 2018).

Kumar et al. (2019) states that using Blockchain, clustering, and classification machine learning, a novel framework for malware detection with Internet of Things (IoT) devices in the healthcare industry was suggested. Using clustering and classification techniques, the machine learning system automatically gathers information about dangers and stores it in Blockchain. The dataset used includes 6192 good and 5560 bad apps that were gathered from the Chinese App Store and the Google Play Store. For evaluation measurement, they acquire true positive and false positive rates as well as classification precision. The disadvantages of the solution include its inability to handle such concealment techniques and features while constructing Apks using Dex2jar.

Akarca et al. (2019) explored regulatory frameworks for health data management, patient rights, cybersecurity, and provider-centric perspectives in. They were able to use blockchain technology to streamline hospital operations and minimise transaction costs by utilising smart contracts. to increase patient rights management, health record processing, and defence against Ransomware attacks They provided regulatory

Figure 4. Ransomware attacks in 2022
Source: crowdstrike.com

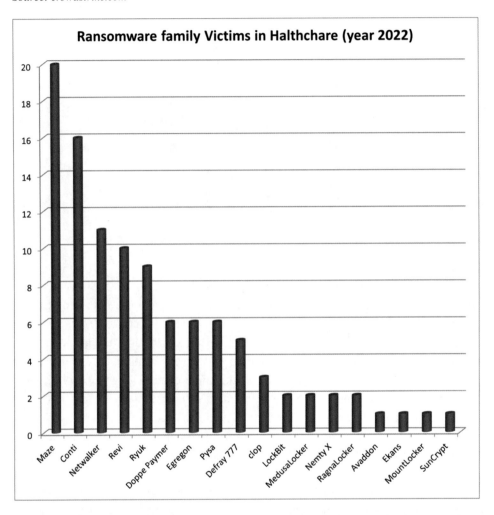

frameworks that use Blockchain technology to optimise healthcare practises. They reduced their processing costs by utilising smart contracts.

The authors of Akcora et al. (2019) proposed an effective and manageable data analytics methodology to automatically detect new risky locations in a Ransomware family. Using a topological data analysis-based technique and innovative Blockchain graph-related features, they showed that the suggested methodology delivers noticeably gains in precision and recall for Ransomware transaction identification when compared to current heuristic-based approaches. As a result, it enables automated Ransomware detection. The collection is a compilation of datasets from 27 different ransomware subtypes. However, the results of their study might have been improved by combining their methodology with other approaches and adding intelligence data to improve forecast accuracy.

The majority of people consider machine learning to be one of today's most breakthrough technologies (ML). Machine learning is used to develop algorithms capable of learning from data. The goal of machine learning is to find patterns in data and draw valuable conclusions from them. ML may be applied to health data to build reliable risk models, locate Ransomware malware, and apply deep learning techniques (Jabbar, 2021).

Reddy et al. (2021) outlines an innovative approach to ransomware detection that solely use hexacodes, ignores opcodes, and makes use of machine learning classifiers. Two functional strategies are the Information Benefit (IG) and Gain Ratio (GR) methodologies. They discovered that RF-IG had a significant statistical effect. Deep learning methods as classifiers and shell-based feature discovery methods are both advised for use with Hexacodes features. A paper word matrix might also be created by substituting the hex term frequency inverse document frequency (TF-IDF) values for the frequency. It is possible to use the hex reverse document frequency (TF-IDF) values.

Users of software and systems used in medical can identify the abnormality, according to Thamer and Alubady (2021)'s authors. The risk index was calculated by the person who exhibited these behaviours based on how closely they mirrored normative behaviour. Once the risk value has been evaluated in real-time, the device may challenge Multi-Factor Authentication (MFA), refuse access to risky events, or access a low-risk event during a login event. In order to move from reactive to proactive data management, applications for artificial intelligence (AI) and machine learning (ML) take into account the clinical context of each access and adopt a comprehensive perspective of how Electronic Healthcare Recorder (EHR) users interact with patient data. This can improve healthcare industry cybersecurity by immediately recognising behavioural issues.

The authors of Hirano and Kobayashi (2019) disclosed a machine learning model for learning based on ransomware detection. They looked into the characteristics of a real-time forensic hypervisor called "Way back Visor access patterns." They also used data from hardware I/O logs that was cinematic in nature to identify Ransomware from safe programmes that closely resemble Ransomware. There have been developed machine learning models such as Random Forest, Support Vector Machine, and K-Nearest Neighbors. The result of their research employing five-dimensional characteristics was a 98% Fmeasurement score. The development and evaluation of machine learning models took into account the aforementioned factors.

RANSOMWARE ATTACKS IN HEALTHCARE PRESENT PROBLEMS

Table 2. Technique and pros and cons of AI and blockchain technology

Ref.	Technique	Purpose	Pros	Cons
(Kumar et al., 2019) (Alhawi et al., 2018) (Mohammed et al., 2021)	Blockchain and Artificial intelligence	Detecting ransomware on Android IoT devices should be improved.	A framework can identify ransomware more accurately and with fewer false-positive and false-negative rates.	Its inability to deal with such hidden strategies and features while building Apk using Dex2jar.
(Angst & Block, 2017) (Akarca et al., 2019)	Blockchain, Smart Contract	Enabling patients to offer better health data collection, utilisation, and sharing would enhance healthcare practises.	supporting the management of health information while keeping in mind patient rights, governing laws, and cyber security	Issues with Scalability and Storage for Nodes and Networks Needing More Bandwidth and power consumption
(Akcora et al., 2019)	Blockchain-related graph characteristics	The blockchain technology has many uses and applications are more security to protect healthcare	Effective and manageable data analytics framework for automatically detecting new malicious addresses in a ransomware family	Difficult to understand Ransomware address detection after the ransom is paid
(Reddy et al., 2021) (Hirano & Kobayashi, 2019) (Maniath et al., 2017)	Machine Learning	Extract data- driven rules of Hexacode based Ransomware	Detect & prevent Ransomware only from Hexacodes using ML	High Level of Error Susceptibility
(Thamer & Alubady, 2021) (Al-Jaija et al., 2020)	Artificial Intelligence and Machine Learning	Greater protection for organizations and patients from Ransomware	Identify the abnormality in healthcare systems	Susceptible to errors
(Thamer & Alubady, 2021) (Alhawi et al., 2018)	Machine learning, Domain Generation Algorithm	Provide security for Patient data from EMRs	Multiclassifier intrusion detection system, detect operation of Ransomware in case of locky	The acute lack of Ransomware datasets was a key problem

CONCLUSION

Cybersecurity in health care is now universally recognised as a serious patient safety risk, as evidenced by multiple recent examples of how hacks hurt healthcare organisations. This study found that healthcare organisations have made some progress toward using AI and blockchain to improve accuracy and safety cybersecurity inside organisations globally, but cybersecurity maturity is still uneven and has to be improved in almost every environment. In order to improve cybersecurity in healthcare and to better comprehend the larger healthcare and legislative contexts, it is important to scale up preparatory efforts in this area and to adopt policies.

REFERENCES

Akarca, D., Xiu, P. Y., Ebbitt, D., Mustafa, B., Al-Ramadhani, H., & Albeyatti, A. (2019, June). Blockchain secured electronic health records: patient rights, privacy and cybersecurity. In *2019 10th International Conference on Dependable Systems, Services and Technologies (DESSERT)* (pp. 108-111). IEEE.

Akbanov, M., Vassilakis, V. G., & Logothetis, M. D. (2019). Ransomware detection and mitigation using software-defined networking: The case of WannaCry. *Computers & Electrical Engineering*, 76, 111–121. doi:10.1016/j.compeleceng.2019.03.012

Akcora, C. G., Li, Y., Gel, Y. R., & Kantarcioglu, M. (2019). *BitcoinHeist: Topological data analysis for ransomware detection on the bitcoin blockchain.* arXiv preprint arXiv:1906.07852.

Al-Haija, Q. A., McCurry, C. D., & Zein-Sabatto, S. (2020, September). Intelligent self-reliant cyber-attacks detection and classification system for IoT communication using deep convolutional neural network. In *International Networking Conference* (pp. 100-116). Springer.

Al-rimy, B. A. S., Maarof, M. A., & Shaid, S. Z. M. (2018). Ransomware threat success factors, taxonomy, and countermeasures: A survey and research directions. *Computers & Security*, 74, 144–166. doi:10.1016/j.cose.2018.01.001

Alhawi, O. M., Baldwin, J., & Dehghantanha, A. (2018). Leveraging machine learning techniques for windows ransomware network traffic detection. In *Cyber threat intelligence* (pp. 93–106). Springer. doi:10.1007/978-3-319-73951-9_5

Almashhadani, A. O., Kaiiali, M., Sezer, S., & O'Kane, P. (2019). A multi-classifier network-based crypto ransomware detection system: A case study of locky ransomware. *IEEE Access : Practical Innovations, Open Solutions*, 7, 47053–47067. doi:10.1109/ACCESS.2019.2907485

Angst, C. M., Block, E. S., D'Arcy, J., & Kelley, K. (2017). When do IT security investments matter? Accounting for the influence of institutional factors in the context of healthcare data breaches. *Management Information Systems Quarterly*, 41(3), 893–A8. doi:10.25300/MISQ/2017/41.3.10

Cimpanu, C. (2020). *Hackers preparing to launch ransomware attacks against hospitals arrested in Romania.* ZDNet. https://www. zdnet. com/ article/ hackers-preparing-to-launch-ransomware-attacks-against-hospitals-arrested-in-romania/

Dempster, B., & Eaton-Lee, J. (2006). *Configuring IPCop Firewalls: Closing Borders with Open Source.* Packt Publishing Ltd.

Donnan, S. (2019). *Bloomberg-Are you a robot?* Bloomberg. com.

El Hajal, G., Yves, D. U. C. Q., & Börcsök, J. (2019, October). Designing and validating a cost effective safe network: application to a PACS system. In *2019 Fifth International Conference on Advances in Biomedical Engineering (ICABME)* (pp. 1-4). IEEE. 10.1109/ICABME47164.2019.8940252

Foley, L., Foley, L., Hoffman, S. K., McGinley, T. G., Barney, K., Nelson, C., & Tosouni, A. (2003). *Identity theft: The aftermath 2003.* Gartner Research Group.

Gautam, T., & Jain, A. (2015). Analysis of brute force attack using TG — Dataset. *2015 SAI Intelligent Systems Conference (IntelliSys)*, 984-988. 10.1109/IntelliSys.2015.7361263

Georgiadou, A., Mouzakitis, S., & Askounis, D. (2021). *Designing a cyber-security culture assessment survey targeting critical infrastructures during covid-19 crisis.* arXiv preprint arXiv:2102.03000.

Ghafir, I., Prenosil, V., Hammoudeh, M., Baker, T., Jabbar, S., Khalid, S., & Jaf, S. (2018). BotDet: A system for real time botnet command and control traffic detection. *IEEE Access: Practical Innovations, Open Solutions*, 6, 38947–38958. doi:10.1109/ACCESS.2018.2846740

He, Y. (2021). *Health Care Cybersecurity Challenges and Solutions Under the Climate of COVID-19: Scoping Review.* PubMed Central. www.ncbi.nlm.nih.gov/pmc/articles/PMC8059789

He, Y., Aliyu, A., Evans, M., & Luo, C. (2021). Health care cybersecurity challenges and solutions under the climate of COVID-19: Scoping review. *Journal of Medical Internet Research*, 23(4), e21747. doi:10.2196/21747 PMID:33764885

Hedayati, A. (2012). An analysis of identity theft: Motives, related frauds, techniques and prevention. *Journal of Law and Conflict Resolution*, 4(1), 1–12.

Hirano, M., & Kobayashi, R. (2019, October). Machine learning based ransomware detection using storage access patterns obtained from live-forensic hypervisor. In *2019 sixth international conference on internet of things: Systems, Management and security (IOTSMS)* (pp. 1-6). IEEE. 10.1109/IOTSMS48152.2019.8939214

Jabbar, M. A. (2021). Breast cancer data classification using ensemble machine learning. *Engineering and Applied Science Research, 48*(1), 65–72.

Karapapas, C., Pittaras, I., Fotiou, N., & Polyzos, G. C. (2020, May). Ransomware as a service using smart contracts and IPFS. In *2020 IEEE International Conference on Blockchain and Cryptocurrency (ICBC)* (pp. 1-5). IEEE. 10.1109/ICBC48266.2020.9169451

Kumar, R., Zhang, X., Wang, W., Khan, R. U., Kumar, J., & Sharif, A. (2019). A multimodal malware detection technique for Android IoT devices using various features. *IEEE Access : Practical Innovations, Open Solutions, 7*, 64411–64430. doi:10.1109/ACCESS.2019.2916886

Le, Y., Wang, Z. J., Quan, Z., He, J., & Yao, B. (2018, July). ACV-tree: A New Method for Sentence Similarity Modeling. IJCAI, 4137-4143.

Maher, B. S. (2011). Some thoughts on health care exchanges: Choice, defaults, and the unconnected. *Connecticut Law Review, 44*, 1099.

Maniath, S., Ashok, A., Poornachandran, P., Sujadevi, V. G., AU, P. S., & Jan, S. (2017, October). Deep learning LSTM based ransomware detection. In *2017 Recent Developments in Control, Automation & Power Engineering (RDCAPE)* (pp. 442-446). IEEE.

Mohammed, R., Alubady, R., & Sherbaz, A. (2021). Utilizing blockchain technology for IoT-based healthcare systems. *Journal of Physics: Conference Series, 1818*(1), 012111. doi:10.1088/1742-6596/1818/1/012111

Mohurle, S., & Patil, M. (2017). A brief study of wannacry threat: Ransomware attack 2017. *International Journal of Advanced Research in Computer Science, 8*(5), 1938–1940.

Mujeye, S. (2022). Ransomware: To Pay or Not to Pay? The results of what IT professionals recommend. In *2022 The 5th International Conference on Software Engineering and Information Management (ICSIM)* (pp. 76-81). Academic Press.

Oso, A. A., Adefurin, A., Benneman, M. M., Oso, O. O., Taiwo, M. A., Adebiyi, O. O., & Oluwole, O. (2019). Health insurance status affects hypertension control in a hospital based internal medicine clinic. *International Journal of Cardiology. Hypertension, 1*, 100003. doi:10.1016/j.ijchy.2019.100003 PMID:33447737

Reddy, B. V., Krishna, G. J., Ravi, V., & Dasgupta, D. (2021). *Machine learning and feature selection based ransomware detection using hexacodes. In evolution in computational intelligence*. Springer.

Runciman, B. (2020). Cybersecurity report 2020. *Itnow*, *62*(4), 28–29. doi:10.1093/itnow/bwaa103

Schmitz, P., Hildebrandt, J., Valdez, A. C., Kobbelt, L., & Ziefle, M. (2018). You spin my head right round: Threshold of limited immersion for rotation gains in redirected walking. *IEEE Transactions on Visualization and Computer Graphics*, *24*(4), 1623–1632. doi:10.1109/TVCG.2018.2793671 PMID:29543179

Sittig, D. F., & Singh, H. (2016). A socio-technical approach to preventing, mitigating, and recovering from ransomware attacks. *Applied Clinical Informatics*, *7*(02), 624–632. doi:10.4338/ACI-2016-04-SOA-0064 PMID:27437066

Thamer, N., & Alubady, R. (2021). A Survey of Ransomware Attacks for Healthcare Systems: Risks, Challenges, Solutions and Opportunity of Research. *International Journal on Computer Science and Engineering*, *6*(1), 80–85.

Thamer, N., & Alubady, R. (2021). A Survey of Ransomware Attacks for Healthcare Systems: Risks, Challenges, Solutions and Opportunity of Research. *1st Babylon International Conference on Information Technology and Science (BICITS)*, 210-216. 10.1109/BICITS51482.2021.9509877

Thamer, N., & Alubady, R. (2021, April). A Survey of Ransomware Attacks for Healthcare Systems: Risks, Challenges, Solutions and Opportunity of Research. In *2021 1st Babylon International Conference on Information Technology and Science (BICITS)* (pp. 210-216). IEEE.

Usak, M., Kubiatko, M., Shabbir, M. S., Viktorovna Dudnik, O., Jermsittiparsert, K., & Rajabion, L. (2020). Health care service delivery based on the Internet of things: A systematic and comprehensive study. *International Journal of Communication Systems*, *33*(2), e4179. doi:10.1002/dac.4179

Venter, I. M., Blignaut, R. J., Renaud, K., & Venter, M. A. (2019). Cyber security education is as essential as "the three R's". *Heliyon*, *5*(12), e02855. doi:10.1016/j.heliyon.2019.e02855 PMID:31872107

Wani, A., & Revathi, S. (2020). Ransomware protection in IoT using software defined networking. *Iranian Journal of Electrical and Computer Engineering*, *10*(3), 3166–3175.

Yamany, B. (2022). *A New Scheme for Ransomware Classification and Clustering Using Static Features*. MDPI. www.mdpi.com/2079-9292/11/20/3307/html

Zakus, D., Bhattacharyya, O., & Wei, X. (2014). Health systems, management, and organization in global health. In *Understanding Global Health* (2nd ed.). McGrawHill. https://accessmedicine.mhmedical.com/content.aspx?bookid=710& sectionid=46796921

Chapter 5
Secure Data Sharing Using Revocable-Storage Identity-Based Encryption

Muthumanikandan Vanamoorthy
Vellore Institute of Technology, Chennai, India

ABSTRACT

Distributed computing provides flexible and informative information exchange and brings many benefits to both the general public and individuals. However, because the information often contains the most important data, there is a common lock that allows users to easily reuse cloud host information. Therefore, it is important for users to provide cryptographically enhanced access control to shared resources. Personality-based encryption is, for example, a promising encryption approach for building smart data sharing systems. Anyway, access to management is not a versatile solution. In such cases, if your permission is revoked from the database, it must be completely revoked from the cloud server, and you will not be able to retrieve your information once it has been revoked. It has many features of realizability, usefulness, and effectiveness and thus shows the correlation that shows the proposed method diagram used to build a practical and intelligent data provider structure.

INTRODUCTION

Data sharing has become a ubiquitous aspect of modern life, however, with increased connectivity and data exchange comes with increased security risks. To mitigate these risks, various encryption techniques have been developed to protect sensitive information. One such technique is Revocable-Storage Identity-Based Encryption (RS-IBE). RS-IBE is a powerful encryption mechanism that enhances the security of shared data by combining the advantages of Identity-Based Encryption (IBE) with the ability to revoke access to encrypted data. Secure Data Sharing using Revocable-

DOI: 10.4018/978-1-6684-6646-9.ch005

Storage Identity-Based Encryption (RS-IBE) is a cutting-edge encryption technique that enhances the security of shared data. It combines the benefits of Identity-Based Encryption (IBE) with the ability to revoke access to encrypted data, ensuring that only authorized users have access to sensitive information. RS-IBE allows for secure data sharing across multiple platforms and devices while maintaining the privacy and confidentiality of the shared information. IBE is a type of public key encryption that uses a user's identity, such as an email address, as the public key. This eliminates the need for a public key infrastructure, making it a more efficient and scalable solution for data encryption. RS-IBE extends IBE by incorporating the capability to revoke access to encrypted data, ensuring that only authorized users have access to the sensitive information. RS-IBE is particularly useful for secure data sharing across multiple platforms and devices, as it enables the encrypted data to be stored in a central location, such as a cloud storage provider. In the event that a user's authorization is revoked, the encrypted data remains secure and can only be accessed by authorized users. In this computational data storage a computer process which offers huge task that hold massive storage capacity with low value. This provides the customers who can obtain the service they require despite the time or location, and it does so across various domain, bringing considerable ease to cloud users. Data services in various domain applications among which it has many services provided by cloud computing and can deliver an effective and convenient process which distributes information that is shared across the network and provides significant advantage for the users. Moreover, it is vulnerable to a number of security issues, which are among cloud customers' primary concerns. Users may be reluctant because outsourced data typically contains efficient and important informative data. Second, the data is shared commonly and carried out in an extended atmosphere, rendering data services susceptible to cyber-attack. Moreover, the cloud server itself may be used to illegally profit from the data of its users. Finally, shared data is not in fixed process. Which is when the user authentication has expelled, they will not be able to access previously and subsequent shared data. As a result, when information is delivered to a data hostile in which the user will be able to manage the data in which users who are currently permitted to share the information. Confidentiality and backward secrecy can be provided by a data sharing system. Moreover, the methodology of decrypt and rewrite the encrypted data which ensures safety and security . This comes with other hurdles . Indeed users or the people who authorize require the key decrypt-then encrypt the process that involves the use of users' private key information, making the entire shared data through which it forms threats. The data provider must frequently repeat to do decrypt-encrypt process while uploading file procedure to make sure the encrypted message of the shared data up to date. This method has a high communication and compute cost, rendering it difficult and not reasonable for customers in limited and computed and warehouse capacity.

LITERATURE SURVEY

This survey focuses on online social network connections. This is often related to actual interactions and can be used to predict trust between individuals. We suggest using these connections to build a continuous "social cloud" that allows people to use their knowledge resources within networking sites. In addition, you can use the environment modification techniques created to create internet structures for long-term collaboration with less privacy and security concerns than traditional cloud environments. Social markets are unusual in that they combine social and economic standards to facilitate trading. Used to facilitate trading (Chard, K et.al., 2011).

Network management is a challenge for users with limited access to information, as users no longer have direct control over offsite data. However, users can use the server without worrying about checking the integrity of the server. As a result, releasing open source data is an important task for customers. Customers may be able to rely on unauthorized users to validate the data they share together, while remaining cost-effective. Because deployment is safe for unauthorized users, auditing methods should introduce data security without misunderstandings about information protection and eliminate interaction with onsite consumers (Wang, C et.al., 2011).

A procedure is suggested to verify the authenticity of the series from unauthorized users before saving the data (Libert, B et.al., 2009). This approach includes access control to ensure that only authorized personnel can encrypt data. Users can add, modify, and view data stored on the network, and the system protects them from replay attacks. It also discusses access control issues (Ruj, S et.al., 2013).

This is a detailed analysis of the information distributed to achieve the interests of a particular customer. Data is shared by a wide range of groups and individuals, but there are several factors to consider. Ring signatures are a convenient way to detect unauthorized data information. This allows unauthorized users to authenticate their information. This information can be maintained or evaluated in the cloud (Huang, X et.al., 2014).

In cloud storage, data sharing is a crucial feature. Via this post, we'll teach you how to send information to other onsite in a secure, efficient, and flexible manner (Chen, J et.al., 2012). It provide a new open source key crypto technique that generate cypher text, allowing for correct decoded techniques in delegation to any cypher text. The breakthrough is a collection of secret information that can be combined to form a secret system. In a holder of the privacy key for consistent size for key in cloud storage flexibility in cypher text sets, while the decoded file stay private. It's a little a technique key that is easily shared or saved on a a small amount of safe storage. We provide reliability and security over the analysis (Chu, C. K et.al., 2013).

Any feature, regardless of whether the user has been deleted from the database. With a traditional PKI setup, this is a big open problem. However, IBE-related withdrawal procedures have been studied only to a limited extent (Seo, J. H et.al., 2013). The most practical approach would require the recipient to call a concession while encrypting the data to change the private key on a regular basis. Keep in mind that this strategy cannot be extended well as the keys change as the number of users increases. Our method is provable, secure and based on flexible IBE primitives and binary graph databases (Boldyreva, A et.al., 2008).

It can be canceled and can hardly be changed by anything that deals only with the IBE expiration method. Until recently, best practice was to add time to the ID during encoding. As a result, unauthorized users must provide the decrypted key due to frequent interruptions, which causes authentication issues. Unfortunately, secure information can be asserted in certain identity states (Yang, K et.al., 2012).

However, encrypted and updated keys are still a difficult problem. The research we conducted provides a positive solution to the problem of efficiency of involuntary dismissal. A technique that allows you to delegate both lock and decryption permissions for a user. Certain eras of the cloud are coming to an end, whether or not the user's permission has already been revoked (Phan, D. H et.al.,2013). If the user's credentials are removed in the next few years, they will not be able to decrypt messages encrypted with the full privacy key. The new scheme offers significant communication and computational efficiency benefits, especially when compared to interacting with unauthorized users for a period of time (Liang, K et.al., 2014).

The research we conducted provides a positive solution to the problem of efficiency of involuntary dismissal. A technique that allows you to delegate both lock and decryption permissions for a user. Certain eras of the cloud are coming to an end, whether or not the user's permission has already been revoked. If the user's credentials are removed in the next few years, they will not be able to decrypt messages encrypted with the full privacy key. The new scheme offers significant communication and computational efficiency benefits, especially when compared to interacting with unauthorized users for a period of time (Ramesh, R et.al., 2017). Software Defined Networks play a major in providing security in an efficient manner (Vanamoorthy, M et.al., 2020). An alternative approach for hadoop based frame work using C++ was proposed which also has the possibility to improve security (Srinivasakumar, V et.al., 2022).

PROBLEM DEFINITION

Unauthorized users may be advised to obtain sensitive keys from the key authority on a regular basis as a common undoable method. The solution is unstable, so unrevoked users need to get key authentication to perform linear work. You must use a secure channel to send a new key and approve key authentication.

- Franklin and Bowney first proposed a specific undoable method.
- Goyal, Boldyreva, and Kumar have developed ways to implement certain undoable methods. They used identification and a systematic approach reduced the difficulty of being revoked by a limited number of clients.

PROPOSED METHOD

The proposed system of "Secure Data Sharing using Revocable-Storage Identity-Based Encryption (RS-IBE)" aims to provide a secure and efficient solution for sharing sensitive information. This system leverages the benefits of Identity-Based Encryption (IBE) and combines them with the ability to revoke access to encrypted data. The system employs RS-IBE as the encryption mechanism to secure the shared data. RS-IBE uses a user's identity as the public key, eliminating the need for a public key infrastructure and making it a more scalable solution for data encryption. In addition, the system incorporates the ability to revoke access to encrypted data, ensuring that only authorized users have access to sensitive information. The proposed system enables secure data sharing across multiple platforms and devices. The encrypted data can be stored in a central location, such as a cloud storage provider, making it accessible to authorized users. In the event that a user's authorization is revoked, the encrypted data remains secure and can only be accessed by authorized users. The proposed system addresses the security risks associated with data sharing by providing a secure and efficient solution for data encryption and access control. The use of RS-IBE ensures the confidentiality and privacy of the shared information, while the ability to revoke access to encrypted data ensures that only authorized users have access to sensitive information.

- It is presented in natural way for a particular technique and security techniques that goes with it.
- We demonstrate an RSIBE concrete structure. The proposed system can concurrently provide confidentiality and backward/forward2 secrecy. Figure 1 has the following components.
    1. Key Generation: A trusted Key Generation Center (KGC) generates a secret key for each user and publishes a public key.
    2. Identity-Based Encryption: The data owner encrypts the data with the recipient's public key and stores it in a remote storage.
    3. Revocation: In case a user's identity is compromised, the KGC can revoke their secret key and issue a new one, rendering any previous encrypted data inaccessible to the attacker.
    4. Data Access: To access the encrypted data, the recipient sends a request to the data owner, who then sends the encrypted data to the recipient along with a

session key encrypted with the recipient's secret key. The recipient uses their secret key to decrypt the session key and then use it to decrypt the data.

5. Security: The proposed method provides secure data sharing as the data is encrypted using identity-based encryption, which is secure against chosen ciphertext attacks, and the key revocation mechanism ensures that even if a user's identity is compromised, the attacker cannot access their encrypted data.

6. Efficiency: The proposed method also provides efficient data access as the recipient does not need to contact the KGC for every access, as the session key is encrypted using the recipient's secret key, which they can use to decrypt the data.

SYSTEM ARCHITECTURE

Figure 1. System architecture

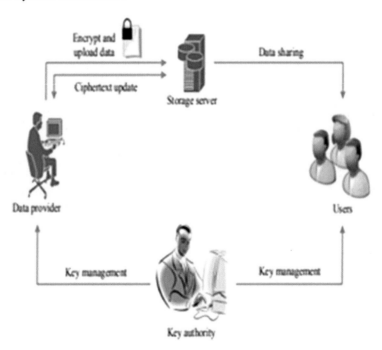

EXPERIMENTAL SETUP

In this experiment we have used Html, CSS, bootstrap for front end and for backend we have used PHP. The System requirements we have used here is Windows 10.

The Software Tools and Language used are Web Development, Visual Studio, Embedded Java Script.

IMPLEMENTATION

The project is done on visual studio platform and connected to local host(php) where it runs on the server and if you give the node app.js on the terminal in visual studio and the file connect to localhost.

Once you connected the localhost and then open the xampp and click the start button, it connects the database in the backend and runs on the localhost.

Enter the localhost:3000 to the chrome browsers so that the page can be viewed clearly. Once you open the main page of the project it will contains a detail view of project.

The other is also known as home page where there consists of

- Home
- Data Provider
- Data User
- Key Auditor

Data Provider

The work of the data provider is that the data supplier selects the user with whom he wanted to share the data and whom the data can be shared across the internet and by the encoded information by using the multiple user's he signifies and send's the shared data in cypher text.In correspondence which the third parties cannot be exposed to the data.

Data User

The data user module is designed in such a way that new users must first register before logging in for authentication. The Cloud will enable the option to search for files. Then, for sending the request to auditor for file access, data user functionality is created. He or she can access the File after receiving the decrypt key from the auditor. The file can also be downloaded by the data user. The user logs out of the session once the process is completed.

Key Auditor

The auditor will log in to the auditor's page. The user will look into any of the above person's pending requests. They are generating a privacy key in encrypting the privacy key for decrypting accepting to request from an aforesaid individual. The auditor logs out of the session when task is completed.

1. Scalability: The proposed method can be improved to handle a large number of users and data owners efficiently. This can be achieved by implementing efficient algorithms for key management and revocation.
2. Privacy-Preserving Revocation: The key revocation mechanism in the proposed method may reveal information about the revoked user's identity. Research can be done to develop a privacy-preserving revocation mechanism that does not compromise the user's privacy.
3. Dynamic Data Ownership: In the proposed method, the data owner is fixed, but in some scenarios, the data owner may change dynamically. Future work can explore the development of a method for revocable-storage identity-based encryption that supports dynamic data ownership.
4. Cloud-Based Implementation: The proposed method can be implemented in a cloud environment to allow for secure data sharing in cloud storage. Further research can be conducted to optimize the performance and security of the proposed method in a cloud environment.
5. Integration with Access Control: The proposed method focuses on encryption-based security, but access control can also play a significant role in secure data sharing. Future work can integrate access control mechanisms with the proposed method to provide a comprehensive solution for secure data sharing.

RESULTS

Figure 2, Figure 3, Figure 4, and Figure 5 represent the results obtained from the proposed storage identity based encryption.

CONCLUSION

Cloud storage has many benefits, including increased storage capacity, reduced costs, reduced direct service costs, and improved storage reliability. Within this IT ecosystem, setting up an overall repository of information stored in databases

Figure 2. Audit log comparison

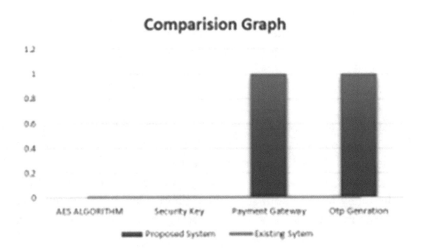

Figure 3. Secure methods

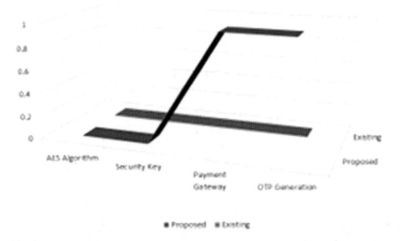

is a major obstacle. Most of this article focuses on security and privacy issues, as well as many strategies that are working in today's public cloud. In addition, a number of strategies help enhance the protection of stored data and ensure the anonymity of information. Infrastructure was the dominant innovation for technical applications.

In conclusion, the proposed method for secure data sharing using revocable-storage identity-based encryption is a secure and efficient solution for protecting

Figure 4. Storage based

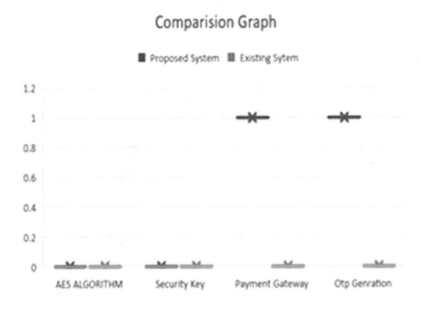

Figure 5. Data sharing

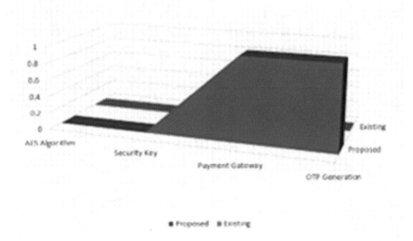

sensitive data. The method leverages the security of identity-based encryption to ensure that the data is protected against unauthorized access, while the key revocation mechanism ensures that even if a user's identity is compromised, the attacker cannot access their encrypted data. The use of session keys encrypted with the recipient's secret key also enhances efficiency by eliminating the need for frequent contact with the Key Generation Center (KGC). Overall, the proposed method provides a strong and practical solution for secure data sharing.

FUTURE WORK

The solutions which accomplish maintain user; renounced clients cannot be able to retrieve their primary data records once they've been renounced, regardless of whether they scheme with an insecure cloud. A future research project will look into ways for a data owner to hold any third party responsible for malicious activities on their data. Another aspect of the inspection is to offer the data owner physical control over the data. Rather than taking responsibility, the data owner can create a large number of access control rules on his data and provide it along with the entrance control method. As a result, every portion can simply use data preserving the enchance the particular strategy. If a component tries to create illegal copies to the data, the starting data of system will be "lock" and data to prevent over the component by avoid using it. The possible future works are:

1. Scalability: The proposed method can be improved to handle a large number of users and data owners efficiently. This can be achieved by implementing efficient algorithms for key management and revocation.

2. Privacy-Preserving Revocation: The key revocation mechanism in the proposed method may reveal information about the revoked user's identity. Research can be done to develop a privacy-preserving revocation mechanism that does not compromise the user's privacy.

3. Dynamic Data Ownership: In the proposed method, the data owner is fixed, but in some scenarios, the data owner may change dynamically. Future work can explore the development of a method for revocable-storage identity-based encryption that supports dynamic data ownership.

4. Cloud-Based Implementation: The proposed method can be implemented in a cloud environment to allow for secure data sharing in cloud storage. Further research can be conducted to optimize the performance and security of the proposed method in a cloud environment.

5. Integration with Access Control: The proposed method focuses on encryption-based security, but access control can also play a significant role in secure data sharing. Future work can integrate access control mechanisms with the proposed method to provide a comprehensive solution for secure data sharing.

REFERENCES

Boldyreva, A., Goyal, V., & Kumar, V. (2008, October). Identity-based encryption with efficient revocation. In *Proceedings of the 15th ACM conference on Computer and communications security* (pp. 417-426). ACM.

Chard, K., Bubendorfer, K., Caton, S., & Rana, O. F. (2011). Social cloud computing: A vision for socially motivated resource sharing. *IEEE Transactions on Services Computing*, 5(4), 551–563. doi:10.1109/TSC.2011.39

Chen, J., Lim, H. W., Ling, S., Wang, H., & Nguyen, K. (2012). Revocable identity-based encryption from lattices. *Information Security and Privacy: 17th Australasian Conference, ACISP 2012, Wollongong, NSW, Australia, July 9-11, 2012 Proceedings*, 17, 390–403.

Chu, C. K., Chow, S. S., Tzeng, W. G., Zhou, J., & Deng, R. H. (2013). Key-aggregate cryptosystem for scalable data sharing in cloud storage. *IEEE Transactions on Parallel and Distributed Systems*, 25(2), 468–477.

Huang, X., Liu, J. K., Tang, S., Xiang, Y., Liang, K., Xu, L., & Zhou, J. (2014). Cost-effective authentic and anonymous data sharing with forward security. *IEEE Transactions on Computers*, 64(4), 971–983. doi:10.1109/TC.2014.2315619

Liang, K., Liu, J. K., Wong, D. S., & Susilo, W. (2014). An efficient cloud-based revocable identity-based proxy re-encryption scheme for public clouds data sharing. *Computer Security-ESORICS 2014: 19th European Symposium on Research in Computer Security, Wroclaw, Poland, September 7-11, 2014 Proceedings*, 19(Part I), 257–272.

Libert, B., & Vergnaud, D. (2009). Adaptive-ID secure revocable identity-based encryption. In *Topics in Cryptology–CT-RSA 2009: The Cryptographers' Track at the RSA Conference 2009, San Francisco, CA, USA, April 20-24, 2009. Proceedings* (pp. 1-15). Springer Berlin Heidelberg. 10.1007/978-3-642-00862-7_1

Phan, D. H., Pointcheval, D., Shahandashti, S. F., & Strefler, M. (2013). Adaptive CCA broadcast encryption with constant-size secret keys and ciphertexts. *International Journal of Information Security*, 12(4), 251–265. doi:10.100710207-013-0190-0

Ramesh, R., & Revathy, N. (2017). Public auditing for shared data with efficient user revocation in the cloud. *International Journal for Advance Research and Development*, 2(5), 184–189.

Ruj, S., Stojmenovic, M., & Nayak, A. (2013). Decentralized access control with anonymous authentication of data stored in clouds. *IEEE Transactions on Parallel and Distributed Systems*, *25*(2), 384–394. doi:10.1109/TPDS.2013.38

Seo, J. H., & Emura, K. (2013). Revocable identity-based encryption revisited: Security model and construction. *Public-Key Cryptography–PKC 2013: 16th International Conference on Practice and Theory in Public-Key Cryptography, Nara, Japan, February 26–March 1, 2013 Proceedings*, *16*, 216–234.

Srinivasakumar, V., Vanamoorthy, M., Sairaj, S., & Ganesh, S. (2022). An alternative C++-based HPC system for Hadoop MapReduce. *Open Computer Science*, *12*(1), 238–247. doi:10.1515/comp-2022-0246

Vanamoorthy, M., & Chinnaiah, V. (2020). Congestion-free transient plane (CFTP) using bandwidth sharing during link failures in SDN. *The Computer Journal*, *63*(6), 832–843. doi:10.1093/comjnl/bxz137

Wang, C., Chow, S. S., Wang, Q., Ren, K., & Lou, W. (2011). Privacy-preserving public auditing for secure cloud storage. *IEEE Transactions on Computers*, *62*(2), 362–375. doi:10.1109/TC.2011.245

Yang, K., & Jia, X. (2012). An efficient and secure dynamic auditing protocol for data storage in cloud computing. *IEEE Transactions on Parallel and Distributed Systems*, *24*(9), 1717–1726. doi:10.1109/TPDS.2012.278

Chapter 6

A Machine Learning–Based Framework for Intrusion Detection Systems in Healthcare Systems

Janmejay Pant
Graphic Era Hill University, India

Rakesh Kumar Sharma
Pal College of Technology and Management, Haldwani, India

Himanshu Pant
Graphic Era Hill University, India

Devendra Singh
Graphic Era Hill University, India

Durgesh Pant
Uttarakhand Open University, Haldwani, India

ABSTRACT

A reliable intrusion detection system is an important key component of healthcare-based systems. Intrusion detection systems are crucial in e-healthcare because patient medical records must be maintained accurately, safely, and secretly. Errors in diagnosis and therapy might result from changing the actual patient data. It is not possible to handle complex data using traditional techniques. Current network requirements cannot be met by diversified intrusion techniques. In addition to the rise in data, attacks are also escalating rapidly. The area of network security is trending when it comes to machine learning techniques. This study aims to develop a novel machine learning framework for detecting attacks.

DOI: 10.4018/978-1-6684-6646-9.ch006

INTRODUCTION

In recent years, there has been a growing need for applications and domains to use the Internet, resulting in more data being moved and more workload on the network. Even though there are several security mechanisms in place, such as the firewall system, an excellent mitigation and protection system is in place. Firewall systems prevent illegal access to systems after transferring information but cannot track surveillance. If a threat is attempted to penetrate it, it will not be able to detect it. For the network to be controlled, intrusion detection systems (Pande, S. et al., 2021) must be deployed. The intrusion was described as posing a threat to resource availability, confidentiality, and integrity that was either brought on by authorized system operators misusing their authority or by unauthorized system operators taking advantage of particular permissions gaps (Kumaar, M. A. et al., 2001). An intrusion detection system has been the subject of many studies in recent years. The Internet has become one of the best tools for gathering information about the modern world. One of the critical elements of education and business and health purposes can be regarded as the Internet. As a result, Internet data transfers need to be safe. One of the main issues in today's world is internet security. It is crucial to develop a system to safeguard the consumers who utilize the data and the data itself because the Internet is constantly under assault. The intrusion detection system (IDS) was created to meet that need. Network administrators modify intrusion detection systems to thwart malicious attempts. To effectively manage security, intrusion detection systems become crucial. The intrusion detection system discovers and reports any infiltration or network abuse attempts. IDS can perform thorough security analysis, detect, and thwart harmful attacks on the network, and maintain normal functioning throughout any hostile outbreak. Due to the need to maintain the accuracy, confidentiality, and high level of security of patient medical records, intrusion systems are essential in e-healthcare. Any modification to the original patient data has the potential to result in inaccuracies in the diagnosis and treatment process. For intrusion detection, the bulk of artificial intelligence-based systems currently in use were trained on outdated repositories, which may result in more false positives and need for a full algorithm retraining to handle new threats. Since intrusion detection systems are frequently out of date as a result of these behaviours, it is particularly difficult to protect patient records in medical systems. Attacks against organizations mostly aim to take private user information. These signs draw attention to a background that is essential for modern cyberattack detection and prevention.

With the increasing demand for healthcare services, hospitals are adopting e-healthcare systems to promptly meet patient needs. These systems allow for the efficient management of Electronic Health Records (EHR) and Patient Records, which contain vital medical data necessary for constructing accurate diagnoses and treatment plans. As a result, hospitals are integrating EHR and Personal Health Records to ensure seamless and efficient healthcare delivery in response to the rising demand. Innovative medical devices and systems have flourished due to the rapid development of the Internet of Things (IoT). Keeping patient records secure and accurate is imperative when using edge devices. Incorrect diagnosis or treatment could result in the patient's death if these details are changed or corrupted. As a result, advanced Intrusion Detection Systems are necessary to ensure cyber-security in healthcare systems. Every intrusion detection system is made to spot suspicious network activity, mark it as an intrusion attempt, and log or block it as such. Currently, most Real-time IDS software uses an approach that relies on rules, such as signatures-based detection, stateful protocol analysis, and statistical packet analysis. The Intrusion Detection System (IDS) primarily classifies requests as either benign or malicious, with benign indicating a regular request and negative indicating an abnormal or intrusive request. In addition to identifying specific attacks, the IDS can also detect DDoS attacks. Despite this, AI-based systems may produce false positives over actual threats due to the backlog of false positives. Additionally, due to class imbalances and attributes included in the training dataset, the algorithms may be biased in favor of specific assaults. Inaccuracy and prejudice in intrusion detection systems, which may misidentify benign attacks or malicious requests, can endanger patient records. IDSs generally fall into two types depending on how they are placed (Iwendi, C et al., 2020) Signature-based IDS and anomaly-based IDS. The approach known as signature-based detection, or misuse detection, is founded on a detection approach as discussed by (Tavallaee et al., n.d.). An attack can be detected using a signature or pattern using misuse detection. The main disadvantage of misuse detection is that it only recognizes known patterns and does not detect unknown attacks. Detecting unidentified attacks is possible by using anomaly detection. Detecting anonymous attacks is possible by using anomaly detection. Anomalies can be found in a variety of ways. To identify the irregularities, different machine learning techniques are used. Using pre-stored rules, the signature-based methodology can distinguish recognized threats from those that are not stored. To capture the system's normal operations and behaviors, it is recommended to create a sample file, and any deviations or abnormalities from these established patterns should be considered as potential evidence of a threat, as proposed by Tsai et al. (2013). It is important to note that network data includes many redundant attributes with no real value. A more challenging aspect is the process of examining all characteristics. Consequently, all IDS functions do not need to be used.

Additionally, certain parts adversely affect the detection system's efficiency. In addition, Grammatikis et al. (2018) seek efficient characteristics. Various techniques, such as flooding, can be used by DDoS attacks to exhaust available resources quickly. There is a greater danger associated with military and medical applications.

RELATED WORK

Two main categories of intrusion detection methodologies are supervised learning and unsupervised learning. An information collection with labels is used in the previous model to model network behaviour. This construct assumes that these behaviours also exist based on normal behaviour. Depending on the deployment mechanism, intrusion detection techniques are either clustered or dispersed. The IDS is usually implemented in a host or a centralized boundary router. Although it offers overhead connectivity, it does not offer a direct connection between the nodes and the IDS. The problem can be resolved by combining computers and storage. However, more capacity is needed for computing and storage. According to the article, there are three intrusion detection methodologies: signatures, anomalies, and specifications. A network operation will be identified as a threat if its signature coincides with that in the repository. Vincent et al. (2010) show that present techniques for identifying assaults are quite effective at doing so, but they are inefficient at spotting new threats and variants of known threats. The network behaves as an anomaly-based network by equating anomaly-based procedures with normal operation. Alarms are triggered by IDS if there is a significant difference between everyday actions and attacks. The use of anomaly-based approaches can be used to identify new threats. However, the guidelines for each requirement are determined explicitly by a human specialist. As Fan et al. (2019) point out, to the fact that this is a time-consuming and particularly prone to error process. Pajouh et al. (n.d.) propose an IDS model consisting of a two-tier classification module and a two-layer reduction dimension. As well as classifying root attacks (U2R) and local distance attacks (R2L), the proposed model can also classify local distance attacks. A linear analysis of discriminations was used for dimensional reduction and portion analysis. As for Naive Bayes and K-nearest neighbor, they both used the two-tier classification point. Kozik et al. (2022) introduced IoT distributed threat identification techniques that utilize cloud and edge computing. However, Zhang et al. (2019) found that model-based cybersecurity solutions for IoT have limited efficiency effects. Consequently, the methodology may have the potential to detect new threat signatures in real-time. It is worth noting that Pahl et al. have solely examined inter-service contact from a machine perspective (Khan et al., 2018). For addressing the issue, we utilized two approaches: k-means and grid-based methodology. Notably, Hasan et al. (2019) reported that five machine learning models proficiently detect IoT anomalies. An artificial neural network (ANN) is a type of neural network that combines elements of logistic regression, support vector machines (SVM), decision trees (DT), and random forests (RF). In related research, Brun et al. (n.d.) have developed an online method for identifying IoT network attacks that utilizes a dense and unexpected neural network to forecast denial of service (DoS) threats. Diro and Chilamkurti (2017) have developed a system for real-time threat identification using distributed fog-to-things and deep learning threat recognition. Additionally, Feng et al. (2017) have implemented an auto-detection encoder in wireless communication. Lopez-Martin et al. (2017) utilize an IDS conditional variation auto-encoder to embed threat marks into the decoder layers for threat detection. Furthermore, Shone et al. (n.d.) proposed a hybrid model that combines deep and shallow research approaches. Specifically, a non-symmetrical deep autoencoder (NDAE) is employed for unsupervised feature learning. The framework incorporates stacked NDAEs and RF methodologies to establish a classification framework.

PROPOSED METHODOLOGY

There are four main sub-sections in this Section. For the implementation of the proposed framework, a discussion of the data set and system configuration is presented in this subsection 1. KNN, Logistic Regression and Random Forest are discussed in subsections 2,3 and 4, respectively.

1. Data Set and System Description

Based on Tavallaee et al. (n.d.), NSL KDD data set is being evaluated. It was built using the assessment software from DARPA'98 that provided the data set of KDD CUP 99 (KDD'99). There are 42 characteristics in this data set (e.g., length, type of protocol, etc. and a classification. Each threat has a feature showing its form. According to Zarpelao et al. (2017), all attacks can be classified as DoS, Study, R2L, U2R, or regular attacks. Currently, Threats like R2L and U2R are not widely used in an entire network and have a low classification in KDD99. As a result of criticism of KDD99 issues in 2009, the NSL-KDD data set was developed (Ng et al.).

During the learning process, it is possible for high-frequency threats to be learned and consequently affect the test results, as noted by Nijim et al. (n.d.), due to the presence of numerous replicated records in the dataset. The experiment was conducted using a Windows 10 machine equipped with 8 GB of RAM and an i5-processor.

Using these data sets is a standard approach to assessing the IDS methodology's effectiveness. A data set comprising 70% training and 30% testing was used for KDD.

2.   K-Nearest Neighbour

K-nearest neighbor uses a variety of distance measurement techniques. Using the K-nearest neighbour, the most frequent class label is assigned to the test sample based on the k number of training data samples nearest to the test sample. There is a simple and nonparametric approach to classifying samples as K-nearest neighbors (Kozik et al., 2022). There is a difference between a K-nearest neighbour and an inductive learner because a K-nearest neighbor is an instance-based learner.

3.   Logistic Regression

Based on the logistic function, logistic regression typically models a dependent variable based on a factual model. Parameter estimation is its primary focus. Logistic regression can be expressed in the following equation. The parameter denoted as βi is based on the value of b. Additionally, x1 and x2 serve as predictors, while p represents the probability of Y being equal to 1, with y being the response variable, as discussed by Mitchell and Chen (2014).

$$l = \log_b \frac{p}{1-p} = \beta_0 + \beta_0 x_1 + \beta_2 x_2$$

4.   Random Forest

Using bootstrapped samples of original training data, random forests are ensembles of trees, as defined by their developer, Breiman. Putting down a vector of inputs in a forest is a good way of classifying a new object. Voting by trees indicates the trees' decision about an object's class. Overall, the trees in the forest, the forest chooses the classification with the most votes.

RESULT ANALYSIS

Our first transformation will be around the attack field. The first step will be to add a column that encodes 'normal' values as 0 and any other matters as 1. A simple binary model that identifies attacks will be built from this as the classifier.

Three machine learning models (KNN, Logistic regression and random forest) are used in the study. The accuracy of KNN and Random Forest classifier is around 99%. Logistic regression has poor accuracy for the given data set.

Figure 1. Demonstration of data set

	duration	protocol_type	service	flag	src_bytes	dst_bytes	land	wrong_fragment	urgent	hot	...	dst_host_diff_srv_rate	dst_host_same_src_port_rate
0	0	udp	other	SF	146	0	0	0	0	0	...	0.60	0.88
1	0	tcp	private	S0	0	0	0	0	0	0	...	0.05	0.00
2	0	tcp	http	SF	232	8153	0	0	0	0	...	0.00	0.03
3	0	tcp	http	SF	199	420	0	0	0	0	...	0.00	0.00
4	0	tcp	private	REJ	0	0	0	0	0	0	...	0.07	0.00

5 rows × 44 columns

dst_host_serror_rate	dst_host_srv_serror_rate	dst_host_rerror_rate	dst_host_srv_rerror_rate	attack	level	attack_flag	attack_map
0.00	0.00	0.0	0.00	normal	15	0	0
1.00	1.00	0.0	0.00	neptune	19	1	1
0.03	0.01	0.0	0.01	normal	21	0	0
0.00	0.00	0.0	0.00	normal	21	0	0
0.00	0.00	1.0	1.00	neptune	21	1	1

Figure 2. Comparison of machine learning models

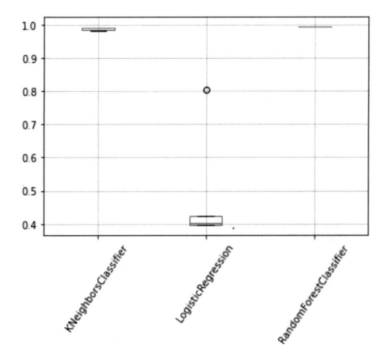

The following measures can be used to assess the effectiveness and bias of machine learning algorithms. The classification performance of a specific method is summarized by a confusion matrix.

Table 1. Confusion matrix for binary classification

	Class 0	Class 1
Class 0	TP	FP
Class 1	FN	TN

The accuracy of the model, equation, or correct rate depends on how well the classification problem is solved.

$$Accuracy = \frac{TP + TN}{TP + TN + FP + FN}$$

CONCLUSION

Intrusion Detection Systems must play a crucial role in an organization's security posture as hospital technology continues to advance and improve. Legally and organizationally, there are too many risks present to ignore them, attacks, vulnerability exploitation, and other dangers. To maintain the integrity of our systems, we must keep an eye on and track these kinds of things. One technique that should be used to

Figure 3. Confusion matrix

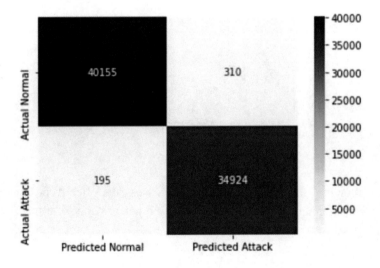

support maintaining this integrity is intrusion detection. In this work, we have used the NSL KDD data set for intrusion detection in health care systems. We compared three crucial machine learning algorithms and found that KNN and Random Forest classifiers provide good accuracy.

REFERENCES

Aly, M., & Khomh, F. (2019, March 27). *Enforcing security in Internet of Things frameworks: A Systematic Literature Review*. https://www.sciencedirect.com/science/article/abs/pii/S2542660518300805

Breiman, L. (2001, October 1). *Random Forests - Machine Learning*. https://link.springer.com/article/10.1023/A:1010933404324

Diro, A. A., & Chilamkurti, N. (2017, September 1). *Distributed attack detection scheme using deep learning approach for Internet of Things*. https://www.sciencedirect.com/science/article/abs/pii/S0167739X17308488

Fan, Y., Zhang, C., Liu, Z., & Qiu, Z. (2019, January 14). *Cost-Sensitive Stacked Sparse Auto-Encoder Models to Detect Striped Stem Borer Infestation on Rice Based on Hyperspectral Imaging*. https://www.sciencedirect.com/science/article/abs/pii/S0950705119300024

Feng, Q., Zhang, Y., Li, C., Dou, Z., & Wang, J. (2017, March 28). Anomaly spectrum detection in wireless communication via deep auto-encoders. *The Journal of Supercomputing*. https://link.springer.com/article/10.1007/s11227-017-2017-7

Fuqaha, A., & Guizani, A. (n.d.). *Internet of Things: A Survey on Enabling Technologies, Protocols, and Applications*. https://ieeexplore.ieee.org/document/7123563

Grammatikis & Moscholios. (2018, November 29). *Securing the Internet of Things: Challenges, threats, and solutions*. https://www.sciencedirect.com/science/article/abs/pii/S2542660518301161?via%3Dihub

Haq, N. F., Onik, A. R., Khan Hridoy, M. A., Rafni, M., Shah, F. M., & Farid, D. M. (2003, March 2). *Application of Machine Learning Approaches in Intrusion Detection System: A Survey*. https://thesai.org/Publications/ViewPaper?Volume=4&Issue=3&Code=IJARAI&SerialNo=2

Hasan, M., & Islam, M. M. (2019, May 20). *Attack and anomaly detection in IoT sensors in IoT sites using machine learning approaches*. https://www.sciencedirect.com/science/article/pii/S2542660519300241

Iwendi, C., Khan, S., Anajemba, J. H., Mittal, M., Alenezi, M., & Alazab, M. (2020, April 30). I *The Use of Ensemble Models for Multiple Class and Binary Class Classification for Improving Intrusion Detection Systems.* https://www.mdpi.com/1424-8220/20/9/2559

Khan, S. H., Hayat, M., Bennamoun, M., & Sohel, F. A. (2018, August 1). *Cost-Sensitive Learning of Deep Feature Representations From Imbalanced Data.* https://pubmed.ncbi.nlm.nih.gov/28829320/

Kozik, R., Choraś, M., Ficco, M., & Palmieri, F. (2022, January 1). *Semantic Scholar is a scalable, distributed machine learning approach for attack detection in edge computing environments.* https://www.semanticscholar.org/paper/A-scalable-distributed-machine-learning-approach-in-Kozik-Chora%C5%9B/eb9d71f3214e793a579d6c3cea9240f882f65d14

Kumaar, M. A., Samiayya, D., Durai Raj Vincent, P. M., Srinivasan, K., Chang, C.-Y., & Ganesh, H. (2001, January 1). A Hybrid Framework for Intrusion Detection in Healthcare Systems Using Deep Learning. *Frontiers.* https://www.frontiersin.org/articles/10.3389/fpubh.2021.824898/full

Lopez-Martin, M., Carro, B., Sanchez-Esguevillas, A., & Lloret, J. (2017, August 26). *Conditional Variational Autoencoder for Prediction and Feature Recovery Applied to Intrusion Detection in IoT.* https://www.mdpi.com/1424-8220/17/9/1967

Mitchell, R., & Chen, I.-R. (2014, April 1). A survey of intrusion detection techniques for cyber-physical systems. *ACM Computing Surveys.* https://dl.acm.org/doi/10.1145/2542049

Nijim, Hisham, Albataineh, Khan, & Rao. (n.d.). *FastDetict: A Data Mining Engine for Predicting and Preventing DDoS Attacks.* Retrieved September 2, 2022, from https://chem.ckcest.cn/Proceeding/Details?id=77324

Olivier, B., Yonghua, Y., & Erol, G. (2018, July 30). *Deep Learning with Dense Random Neural Network for Detecting Attacks against IoT-connected Home Environments.* https://www.sciencedirect.com/science/article/pii/S1877050918311487

Pajouh, H.H., Javidan, R., Khayami, R., Ali, D., & K, C. K. R. (n.d.). *A Two-Layer Dimension Reduction and Two-Tier Classification Model for Anomaly-Based Intrusion Detection in IoT Backbone Networks.* https://ieeexplore.ieee.org/document/7762123

Pande, S., & Khamparia, A. (2021, June 25). *An intrusion detection system for healthcare system using machine and deep learning.* Emerald Insight. https://www.emerald.com/insight/content/doi/10.1108/WJE-04-2021-0204/full/html

Shone, N., Ngoc, T. N., Phai, V. D., & Shi, Q. (n.d.). *A Deep Learning Approach to Network Intrusion Detection.* Retrieved September 2, 2022, from https://ieeexplore. ieee.org/document/8264962

Tavallaee, M., Bagheri, E., Lu, W., & Ghorbani, A. A. (n.d.). *A detailed analysis of the KDD CUP 99 data set.* Retrieved September 1, 2022, from https://ieeexplore. ieee.org/document/5356528

Tesfahun, A., & Bhaskari, D. L. (n.d.). *Intrusion Detection Using Random Forests Classifier with SMOTE and Feature Reduction.* Retrieved September 1, 2022, from https://ieeexplore.ieee.org/document/6701490

Tsai, C. W., Lai, C. F., Chiang, M. C., & Yang, L. T. (2013). Data mining for internet of things: a survey. *IEEE Communications Surveys & Tutorials, 16*(1), 77-97.

Vincent, P., Larochelle, H., Larochelle, H., Bengio, Y., & Manzagol, P. (2010, March 1). Stacked Denoising Autoencoders: Learning Useful Representations in a Deep Network with a Local Denoising Criterion. *The Journal of Machine Learning Research.* https://dl.acm.org/doi/10.5555/1756006.1953039

Wing, Ng, Zeng, & Zhang. (2016, June 21). *Dual autoencoder features for imbalance classification problem.* https://www.sciencedirect.com/science/article/abs/pii/ S0031320316301303

Zarpelao, B. B., Miani, R. S., Kawakami, C. T., & de Alvarenga, S. C. (2017, February 21). *A survey of intrusion detection in Internet of Things.* https://www. sciencedirect.com/science/article/abs/pii/S1084804517300802#!

Zhang, Q., Yang, L., Chen, Z., & Li, P. (2018, January 1). *A survey on deep learning for big data.* https://www.semanticscholar.org/paper/A-survey-on-deep-learning-for-big-data-Zhang-Yang/b7919fadb4c1bf959b1e410463594afacfda7dc6

Chapter 7

Dispute Between Countries, a Corresponding Attack on Cyberspace:
The New National Security Challenge

Siddhardha Kollabathini
Jawaharlal Nehru University, India

ABSTRACT

Today, cyberspace is a fact of daily life, and cyberspace's impact has not bypassed states' national security. Cyberspace, a manmade technological advancement over the past decades, transformed the way economies work around the world, reshaping social interactions and a paradigm shift in politics. Cyberspace being boundaryless, omnipresent across multiple domains, and anarchic has been considered to attack whenever there are any disputes between two countries. In the context described above, a pressing question arises. Cyberspace is not a domain like land, water and air, and it is an environment inhabited by information and knowledge, existing in electronic form. If cyberspace is a mere inhabitation of information and knowledge, why do states want to consider cyberspace as an arena for confrontation in any dispute between countries? This chapter proposes discussing this new phenomenon, looking into the evaluation and analysing aspects of the recent phenomenon.

INTRODUCTION

Over the past decades, cyberspace, a manmade technological advancement, transformed the way economies work worldwide, reshaping social interactions

DOI: 10.4018/978-1-6684-6646-9.ch007

and a paradigm shift in politics. Today cyberspace is a fact of daily life, and it cuts across multiple domains. Cyberspace plays a vital role in atomic energy, space, communications, defence, education, agriculture, manufacture, services, entertainment, and employment generation and in addressing national priorities. Similarly, cyberspace became indispensable in the area of national security and defence. The protection of cyberspace has become a significant challenge to states as cyberspace is intertwined with other warfare domains, namely land, water, air and space.

Interestingly in the realm of the computer networks, state actors are not less in exploiting the incognito, precession impact, cost-effective, minimal human resources requirement characters of cyberspace, which is an informative environment, to achieve national interests. The attacks and threats to national security that are pervasive offline have begun to penetrate the world online. Thus cyberspace has become a new arena of confrontation leading to cyber-insecurity. Such an attack took place in 2007 on Estonia, where Estonia was subjected to systematic distributed attacks for three weeks. The cyber attack crippled the critical information infrastructure of financial centres, banks, parliament, ministries, security and public transport. The cyber attack on Estonia is the first "documented proper cyber attack" and is the beginning of cyber warfare.

Similarly, the attack on Georgia's cyberspace in 2008 changed the threat landscape for all the states that rely on cyberspace. One distinctive characteristic of the cyber attack on Georgia in the above context is – the outbreak of physical hostilities between Georgia and Russia over Abkhazia and South Ossetia landed up in the cyber domain. 'Europe', which became a battlefield for World War One and World War Two, coincidentally became a theatre for confrontation in the cyber domain.

Till the cyber attacks against Estonia 2007 and Georgia 2008, the cyberspace does not have strategic security attire. Pre Estonia 2007 and Georgia 2008 cyber attacks, cyberspace was viewed as a twenty-first-century technological infrastructure, a platform for socio-cultural concepts and a predominant support structure for economic activities. The Estonia and Georgia cyber attacks led to the conclusion that the cyberspace meant to conduct commerce, communicate with the citizens and interface with the critical infrastructure via electronic means can be a battle space and has become a central security concern for governments across the world.

The phenomenon – "whenever there are any disputes between two countries, a corresponding attack on the digital space has been seen" become more common in recent times. The 2010 Stuxnet cyber attack to cripple Iran's nuclear enrichment program; Operation Nitro Zeus 2015 an elaborate plan developed by the US for a cyber attack on Iran, in the event that diplomatic efforts to limit Iran's nuclear program failed and resulted in a military conflict; and, more recently in 2020 the India-China border clash at Galwan valley led to heightened cyber attacks on India by China, evinced the aforementioned phenomenon. In this context, a pressing question arises: Cyberspace is not a domain like land, water and air. It even does not exist like space. In the words of Wing Commander M K Sharma (Indian Air Force): cyberspace is a bio-electronic environment that is literally universal, it exists where there are telephone wires, coaxial cables, fiber-optic lines or electro-magnetic waves. This environment is inhabited by information and knowledge existing in electronic form. If cyberspace is a mere inhabitation of information and knowledge, why do states want to consider cyberspace as an arena for confrontation in any dispute between countries or as an area of strategic importance? Intuitively, the answers lie in analysing cyberspace and cyber security in national security.

Review of Literature

Cyber Space and National Security

There is a fair consensus in the literature that our societies are cyber dependent, and cyber security is a growing matter of national security concern. Therefore *Cyberspace* is crucial in studying from the perspective of security and international relations. Cyberspace constitutes an environment significantly different from other realms of internationally regulated activity (Clemente 2013; Meyer 2015; Kuru 2018). Czosseck and Geers (2009) are of the opinion that each era brings with it new techniques and methods of waging war; while military scholars and experts have mastered land, sea, air and space warfare, the time has come that they have to study the art of cyber war also. They felt that cyberspace is narrowly defined, and the concepts of attack, defence, and security remain unchanged, as do the threats posed by adversary propaganda, espionage, and attack on critical infrastructure. Nye (2010) contrasts with Czosseck and Geers (2009) and defines that the characteristics of cyberspace reduced some of the power differentials among actors, and thus provides a good example of the diffusion of power that typifies the global politics in this century.

Czosseck and Geers (2009) were complemented by M.K. Sharma (2011) and Reveron (2012) by saying that "the concept of cyber capabilities in war are slowly emerging" and sites the incident Russian cyber warriors entering the Georgian Ministry of Defence critical infrastructure in strengthening their argument. Sharma (2011) and Reveron (2012) by their books *Cyber Warfare: The Power of the Unseen; Cyber Warfare and National Security: Is securing Military Networks Enough?;* and *Cyber Space and National Security: Threats, Opportunities and Power in Virtual world,* established a coherent framework for understanding how cyberspace fits within the national security.

Rid (2012), in his comprehensive work *'Cyber war will not take place',* argued that cyber war has never happened in the past, it does not occur in the present, and it is highly unlikely that it will disturb our future. Further, he argued that most of the writers on cyberspace in the context of national security distracted from the real significance of cyber security: cyber attacks are not creating more vectors of violent interaction; instead they make previously violent interactions less violent. Rid (2012), with his analysis, opens a fresh viewpoint that cyberspace is not a domain of military activity; instead, the use of computer networks permeates all other domains of military conflict, land, sea, air and space. Contrarily to Rid (2012), Yates (2013), Lieutenant Commander of US Navy and writer of *Cyber Warfare: An Evolution in Warfare not just War Theory*, asserted that cyber attack in conjugation with the military would rise to the level of national security concerns.

Singer and Friedman (2014) altogether brought a new dimension of the debate cyberspace and national security by means of extensively discussing how it all works in cyberspace, why cyberspace matters and what anyone can do in cyberspace. Green (2015) presented a multidisciplinary analysis of cyber war, and Steed (2015) implanted Greens' analysis by illustrating the strategic implications of cyber war. In their writings, Eun and Abmann (2016) opinioned that cyberspace must be taken into consideration more seriously to have enriched analytical and theoretical understanding of international politics in the digital age. Furthermore, they argued that cyberspace does not have changed the very nature of the war, but cyber warfare indeed will reshape the way in which war begins or is carried out in the near future.

Research Methodology

The proposed qualitative research will be inductive. The research analyses perceptions of cyber security issues through the lens of realism. The central assumptions in realism are that "the state is the primary unit of analysis, the state acts rationally to satisfy its national interests, and power and security are state's core values." Primary and secondary sources will be used in the research. Primary sources will include United Nations, India, European Union, and NATO documents and reports on cyber security. Similarly, the study considers primary sources such as India's, the United States', the European Union's, and NATO's national security policies. This research will also make use of secondary sources such as books, articles, and newspaper clippings.

Discussion

Cyberspace and Cyber Security in National Security

In a short story published in 1982, science fiction writer William Gibson coined the term "cyberspace," and with the introduction of the internet in the 1990s, cyberspace entered the real world. Cyberspace is a term that has yet to be fully defined, despite the fact that it has become an inseparable part of our existence. It established a new environment for information and communication, interactions, conducting business, and developing social media, among other things. As a result, it created a new platform for conflict. There is a healthy debate about whether all technological advancements are valuable in and of themselves, but new technology brings with it new challenges. Indeed, because cyberspace has no boundaries and is anarchic, it has been considered a state entity, and states have developed strategies, weapons, and stratagems in the cyber domain to safeguard their critical infrastructures and defend national security. The impact of cyberspace has not been ignored by states' national security.

Cyberspace constitutes an environment significantly different from other realms of internationally regulated activity. The advent of cyberspace accelerated the military use of cyber capabilities, and simultaneously, the militarization of cyberspace took place due to the lack of convention on cyberspace, and the Western world is the epicentre of these changes. Drek.S.Reveron, in his 2012 work on *"Cyber Space and National Security: Threats, Opportunities, and Power in a Virtual World"*, postulated that, by developing a computer language code, one could be capable enough of cyber attacking the systems anywhere in the world across almost all domains that are connected to computers or networks, and it is highly unlikely to attribute the attack. The following summarized cyber attack incidents might help in better understand the complexity of cyberspace and the concerns surrounding it.

In 2007 a diplomatic row reputed between Russia and Estonia when Estonian authorities moved a monument 'Red Army' from the centre of the capital city, Tallinn, to the outskirts of the town. Estonia, an internet-reliant country, was cyber attacked after the initial unrest. The cyber attack brought down the vast computerized infrastructure of Estonia by what experts in cyber security termed a coordinated "denial of services attack". The devastation was such that Ene Ergma, the Speaker of the Estonian Parliament and a nuclear physics scientist, has made the comparison: "When I look at a nuclear explosion and the explosion that happened in our country in May, I see the same thing." As with nuclear radiation, cyber war can destroy a modem state without drawing blood. At the time, Russia was suspected of the attacks, and Moscow has denied allegations of Russian involvement. The Estonian government denounced the attacks as an unprovoked act of aggression and was unsuccessful in establishing the origin of the cyber attack. However, reports and observations on the Estonian cyber attack incident pointed out that while nationalist fervour on the Russian side certainly played a part in rallying independent hackers, there is a possibility that Russia was involved. Scott Shackelford, Cyber security Program chair, Indiana University, specified the Estonia cyber attack as "the first large scale incident of a cyber assault on a state".

Identically, a computer attack on Georgian websites had started slowly in 2008, weeks before the military confrontation on a territorial dispute over Abkhazia and South Ossetia with Russia. Georgia's prominent websites were defaced, for instance, that of Georgia's National Bank and the Ministry of Foreign Affairs. Noticeably, the Georgia cyber attack was the first case in the cyber security history, where an independent cyber attack has taken place in sync with a conventional military operation.

There is another side to the story; over the years, states have also increased their use of cyber operations to further their national interests. In 2015, for example, the United States developed an elaborate plan code named Nitro Zeus aimed at Iran under the President Obama administration. The project was a strategy to be launched after the Stuxnet 2010 cyber incident, to disable Iran's air defenses, communications systems and crucial parts of its power grid in case the nuclear talks between Iran and *P5 plus one* (UN security council permanent members and Germany) fails. The project was shelved in July 2015 after the nuclear deal struck between Iran

and six other nations. The bloodless, cost-effective, precision impact and incognito characters of cyber attack attained a military perspective. A February 2016 report in 'The New York Times' by David E. Sanger and Mark Mazzetti categorically acknowledged that the states started considering cyber attack as an alternative.

Withal, recently in 2020, the India-China border clash at Galwan valley led to heightened frictions between both countries. The Indian establishment responded by banning Chinese mobile apps, legitimately by invoking the provisions mentioned under 69 A of its Information Technological Act. However, the Ministry of Information

Table 1.

Year	Country	Dispute	Cyber Attack
2007	Estonia	Diplomatic row b/w Estonia and Russia over a monument – "Red Army"	Coordinated Distributed Denial of Service Attack.
2008	Georgia	Physical hostility b/w Georgia and Russia over Abkhazia and South Ossetia.	Distributed Denial of Service Attack.
2010	Iran	Conflict b/w US and Iran over Iran's Natanz uranium enrichment plant - a key part of the nuclear power generation process.	A 500 kilobyte computer worm *"Stuxnet"*, the world's documented first cyber/digital weapon.
2015	Iran	Negotiations b/w P5+1 (US, UK, Russia, France, China, plus Germany) and Iran over Iran's Nuclear program.	Comprehensive cyber attack code name *"Nitro Zeus"*. An elaborate plan developed by US for a cyber attack on Iran.
2020	India	India-China border clash at Galwan valley.	Distributed Denial of Service Attack, and Internet Protocol Hijack.

Source: Compiled by the author from various sources

and Technology, Govt. of India, repudiated the Chinese mobile app ban action in any association with the ongoing tension along the Himalayan border.

Furthermore, the Indian government explicitly stated that the unprecedented decision to prohibit Chinese mobile apps was based on security agency reports that China has been engaged in massive data mining in India and has most likely stolen the personal information of Indian citizens. Following the embargo, China launched over 40,000 cyber attacks on Indian cyber space. The India-China cyber attack incident demonstrates that cyberspace is integrated with or conjugated with a military operation, and the cyber attack provides an advantage.

CONCLUSION

Indeed, consistent with the preceding cyberspace, national security, and cyber security illustration, one can safely extrapolate that, in recent decades, cyberspace has become an integral part of our lives, and it has now become an essential component of national security in the twenty-first century. National security, according to Arnold Wolfers's 1952 article on National Security as an Ambiguous Symbol, is the absence of threat to a society's core values. Following Wolfers's argument, as states and societies increasingly become information societies, the threat to information can be viewed as a threat to the core of these societies. Wolfers's logic holds that cyber security in national security must be taken more seriously in order to understand the various perceptions that underpin security in the cyber era. Furthermore, based on the above mentioned cyber attack incident examples, it is evident that whenever there is a dispute between countries, a cyber-attack has occurred.

REFERENCES

Choucri, N. (2014). *Co-evolution of cyberspace and international relations: New challenges for the social sciences*. Academic Press.

Clemente, D. (2013). *Cyber security and global interdependence: what is critical?* Chatham House.

Czosseck, C., & Geers, K. (Eds.). (2009). *The virtual battlefield: perspectives on cyber warfare* (Vol. 3). IOS Press.

Deibert, R. J., Rohozinski, R., & Crete-Nishihata, M. (2012). Cyclones in cyberspace: Information shaping and denial in the 2008 Russia–Georgia war. *Security Dialogue*, *43*(1), 3–24. doi:10.1177/0967010611431079

Dinu, M. S. (2017). The 5th operational domain and the evolution of NATO's cyber defence concept. *Annals–Series on Military Sciences*, *9*(2), 69–77.

Eriksson, J., & Giacomello, G. (2006). The information revolution, security, and international relations:(IR) relevant theory? *International Political Science Review*, *27*(3), 221–244. doi:10.1177/0192512106064462

Eun, Y. S., & Aßmann, J. S. (2016). Cyberwar: Taking stock of security and warfare in the digital age. *International Studies Perspectives*, *17*(3), 343–360.

Green James, A. (2015). Cyber Warfare A multidisciplinary analysis. Academic Press.

Gupta, A. (2016). Securing Cyberspace: A National Security Perspective. In Securing cyberspace: International and Asian perspectives. Institute for Defence Studies and Analyses.

Koser, M., & Thaver, M. (2020). *In 5 days, over 40,000 Chinese Searches for Vulnerabilities in Indian Cyber space*. https://epaper.indianexpress.com/c/52967213

Kostyuk, N., & Zhukov, Y. M. (2019). Invisible digital front: Can cyber attacks shape battlefield events? *The Journal of Conflict Resolution*, *63*(2), 317–347. doi:10.1177/0022002717737138

Nicolas Mazzucchi, A. D. (2019). *Web wars: Preparing for the next Cyber Crisis – new perspectives on shared security: NATO's next 70 Years, Carnegie Europe*. Available at: https://carnegieeurope.eu/2019/11/28/web-wars-preparing-for-next-cyber-crisis-pub-80420

Nye, J. S. Jr. (2010). *Cyber power*. Harvard Univ Cambridge MA Belfer Center for Science and International Affairs.

everon, D. S. (Ed.). (2012). *Cyberspace and national security: threats, opportunities, and power in a virtual world*. Georgetown University Press.

Rid, T. (2012). Cyber war will not take place. *The Journal of Strategic Studies*, *35*(1), 5–32. doi:10.1080/01402390.2011.608939

Sanger, D. E., & Mazzetti, M. (2016). US had cyberattack plan if Iran nuclear dispute led to conflict. *New York Times, 16*.

Sharma, M. K. (2011). *Cyber Warfare: The Power of the Unseen*. KW Publ.

Singer, P. W., & Friedman, A. (2014). *Cybersecurity: What everyone needs to know*. OUP USA.

Steed, D. (2015). The Strategic Implications of Cyber Warfare. In A. Green James (Ed.), *Cyber Warfare A multidisciplinary analysis*. Library of Congress Cataloging-in-Publication Data. doi:10.4324/9781315761565-5

Stiennon, R. (2015). *There Will Be Cyberwar: b How the Move to Network-Centric Warfighting Set The Stage For Cyberwar*. IT-Harvest Press.

Wolfers, A. (1952). "National security" as an ambiguous symbol. *Political Science Quarterly*, *67*(4), 481–502. doi:10.2307/2145138

Yates, J. A. (2013). *Cyber Warfare: An Evolution in Warfare not Just War Theory*. Marine Corps Command.

Chapter 8

A Review on Application of Reinforcement Learning in Healthcare

Chitra A. Dhawale
P.R. Pote College of Engineering and Management, India

Kritika Anil Dhawale
University of Technology Sydney, Australia

ABSTRACT

We are witnessing the era of data science where data is generating in an exponential manner. This big data is working as fuel to explore the business in every domain and healthcare is not the exception for this. Data analysis and data analytics in collaboration with machine learning techniques are playing an important role in every domain. Supervised and unsupervised approaches in machine learning depends on one shot, exhaustive, and reward output. Reinforcement learning (RL) handles these issues with sequential decision making problems, concurrent evaluation, and feedback methods. RL technique can be a suitable candidate for developing powerful solutions in a variety of healthcare domains. This chapter will focus on the broad applications of RL techniques in healthcare domains, which can be helpful to the researchers with systematic understanding of conceptual information, techniques, and an overview of RL applications in healthcare domains for various types of diseases right from chronic diseases and mental disorder.

INTRODUCTION

We are witnessing the era of data science where data is generating in an exponential manner. This big data is working as fuel to explore the business in every domain

DOI: 10.4018/978-1-6684-6646-9.ch008

and healthcare is not the exception for this. Artificial Intelligence (AI) is playing a master key role in healthcare from the last decade due to its specialty in handling large multimodal data, powerful algorithms and computational models (V. L. Patel, et al, 2009), (S. E. Dilsizian and E. L. Siegel, 2014). Collaborative work of Machine Learning (ML), a subfield of AI, Data Analysis and Data Analytics are playing an important role in every domain (A. E. Johnson, et al, 2016). Supervised and Unsupervised approaches in Machine learning depends on one shot, exhaustive and reward output. Reinforcement Learning (RL) is a machine learning technique that allows an agent to learn by trial and error in an interactive environment using feedback from its own actions and experiences. Reinforcement Learning (RL) handle these issues with sequential decision-making problems, concurrent evaluation and feedback methods. RL technique can be suitable candidate for developing powerful solutions in a variety of healthcare domains (A. Esteva, et al, 2019).

Reinforcement learning (RL), a subdomain of machine learning, has made significant theoretical and technical advances in generalisation, representation, and efficiency in recent years, leading to increased applicability to realworld problems in gaming, robotics control, financial and business management, autonomous driving, natural language processing, computer vision, biological data analysis, and art creation, to name a few. (M. L. Littman, 2018), (V. Mnih, et al, 2015)

REINFORCEMENT LEARNING

Though both supervised and reinforcement learning involve mapping between input and output, reinforcement learning uses incentives and punishments as signals for positive and negative behaviour, unlike supervised learning, which provides the agent with a right set of behaviours for executing a task. Reinforcement learning differs from unsupervised learning in terms of its objectives. In unsupervised learning, the goal is to detect similarities and differences between data points; in reinforcement learning, the goal is to develop an appropriate action model that maximises the agent's total cumulative reward (Shreya Bhatt, 2018).

The main elements of an RL system are:

1. The agent
2. The environment
3. The policy
4. The reward signal

Figure 1. Reinforcement learning system

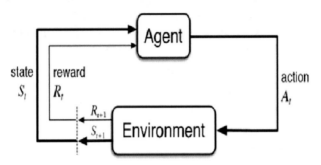

The learning process in which an agent learns action sequences that maximize some notion of reward. The agent, also called an AI agent gets trained in the following manner:

- The agent interacts with the environment and make decisions or choices. For training purpose, the agent is provided with the contextual information about the environment and choices.
- The agent is provided with the feedback or rewards based on how well the action taken by the agent or the decision made by the agent resulted in achieving the desired goal.

The reward signal indicates the subsequent benefit of being in that state while the value function returns the cumulative reward that is projected and obtained from that state forward The purpose of an RL algorithm is to determine the action strategy that maximises the average value extracted from each system state (Ajitesh Kumar, 2022).

REINFORCEMENT ALGORITHMS

RL algorithms can be broadly categorized as model-free and model-based:

Model-free algorithms do not build an explicit model of the environment. They use trial-and-error method that run experiments with the environment using actions and derive the optimal policy from it directly.

Model-free approach either go for value-based or policy-based. Value-based algorithms consider optimal policy to be a direct result of accurately estimating the value function of each state. The agent interacts with the environment to sample state and reward trajectories using a recursive relationship described by the

Bellman equation. The value function of the MDP can be estimated given enough trajectories. Once the value function is known, determining the optimal policy is as simple as acting greedily with respect to the value function at each stage of the process. SARSA and Q-learning are two popular value-based algorithms. Policy-based algorithms, on the other hand, directly estimate the optimal policy without modelling the value function.

They convert the learning problem into an explicit optimization problem by directly parametrizing the policy with learnable weights. The agent, like value-based algorithms, samples state and reward trajectories; however, this information is used to explicitly improve the policy by maximising the average value function across all states. Monte Carlo policy gradient (REINFORCE) and deterministic policy gradient are two popular policy-based RL algorithms (DPG). Policy-based approaches have a high degree of variance, which manifests as instabilities during the training process. Value-based approaches, while more stable, are insufficient for modelling continuous action spaces. The actor-critic algorithm, one of the most powerful RL algorithms, is created by combining the value-based and policy-based approaches. Both the policy (actor) and the value function (critic) in this algorithm are parametrized to allow for effective use of training data while maintaining stable convergence.

Model-based By sampling states, taking actions, and observing the rewards, RL algorithms construct a model of the environment. The model predicts the expected reward and the expected future state for each state and possible action. The first is a regression problem, while the second is a density estimation problem. The RL agent can plan its actions without directly interacting with the environment if it is given a model of the environment. This is similar to a thought experiment that a human might perform when attempting to solve a problem. When the planning process is intertwined with the policy estimation process, the RL agent's ability to learn improves.

APPLICATIONS OF REINFORCEMENT LEARNING IN HEALTHCARE

RL- related models and approaches have been widely applied in healthcare domains since decades ago due to its dominating and unique features against traditional machine learning, statistic learning.

In the early seventy's and eighty's, R.W.Jeliffe along with his coresearchers developed phar- macokinetic/pharmacodynamic (PK/PD) models for applications of DP methods in various pharmacotherapeutic decision making problems (R. W. Jelliffe, et al, 1970).

Schaeffer *et al.* (2005) discussed the benefits and associated challenges of MDP modeling in the context of medical treatment, and reviewed several instances of medical applications of MDPs, such as spherocytosis treatment and breast cancer screening and treatment.

With the vast research work in terms of DL algorithms using reinforcement learning and technical achievements in generalization, representation and efficiency in recent years, RL approaches have been successfully applied in a number of healthcare domains to date. We have categorized the application of RL by categorizing diseases into Chronic,

A.   **Chronic Diseases**

In healthcare domain, Chronic diseases are considered to be most severe public health issue worldwide which causes a considerable portion of death every year (W. H. Organization, 2005). Chronic diseases normally lasts for a long period i.e from three months or more. Due to this long lasting nature, it is expected to require regular clinical observation and medical care.

The widely affecting chronic diseases include endocrine diseases (e.g., diabetes and hyperthyroidism), cardiovascular diseases (e.g., heart attacks and hypertension), various mental illnesses (e.g., depression and schizophrenia), cancer, HIV infection, obesity, and other oral health problems (B. Chakraborty and E. Moodie, 2013).

Long-term treatment of these illnesses is often made up of a sequence of medical intervention that must take into account the changing health status of a patient and adverse effects occurring from previous treatment.

i.   *Cancer*

Cancer is one of the main chronic diseases that causes large number of deaths in world. As per the report of WHO published on 3rd February 2022: Cancer is a leading cause of death worldwide, accounting for nearly 10 million deaths in 2020, or nearly one in six deaths. The most common cancers are breast, lung, colon and rectum and prostate cancers. Around one-third of deaths from cancer are due to tobacco use, high body mass index, alcohol consumption, low fruit and vegetable intake, and lack of physical activity. Cancer-causing infections, such as human papillomavirus (HPV) and hepatitis, are responsible for approximately 30% of cancer cases in low- and lower-middle-income countries. Many cancers can be cured if detected early and treated effectively.

RL methods have been extensively studied in deriving efficient treatment strategies for cancer chemotherapy. Zhao *et al.* (2009) first applied model-free TD method, Q-learning, for decision making of agent dosage in chemotherapy.

The superiority of using continuous dosing treatment over a burst of dosing treatment was also supported by the work (A. Hassani et al., 2010), where naive discrete Q-learning was applied.

More recently, Padmanabhan *et al.* (R. Padmanabhan, et al, 2017) proposed different formulations of reward function in Q-learning to generate effective drug dosing policies for patient groups with different characteristics.

Humphrey (2017) investigated several supervised learning approaches (*Classification And Regression Trees* (CART), random forests, and modified version of *Mutivariate Adaptive Regression Splines* (MARS)) to estimate Q values in a simulation of an advanced generic cancer trial.

Radiopathy is another effective treatment for cancer recovery. Much work on application of RL techniques for automated radiation adaptation protocol is published (M. Feng, et al, 2018).

Agent-based simulation model and Q-learning algorithm proposed by Jalalimanesh *et al.* (2017) is used to optimize dose calculation in radiopathy.

Jalalimanesh *et al.* (2017) extended their research work by proposing a multi-objective Q-Learning algorithm to find the Pareto-optimal solutions for radiotherapy doses, which can erase the tumour with radiation while not impacting normal cells as much as possible. The patient may fade up due to much pain treatment and may drop the treatment in between. This *data censoring problem* (Y. Goldberg and M. R. Kosorok, 2012) complicates the practical use of RL in discovering individualized optimal regimens.

Other studies (Y. M. Soliman, 2014) presented a novel censored-Q-learning algorithm that is tailored for a multi-stage decision problem with a variable number of stages and rewards that are censored survival times.

ii. *Diabetes*

Diabetes is a chronic, metabolic disease characterized by elevated levels of blood sugar, which leads over time to serious damage to the heart, blood vessels, eyes, kidneys and nerves. The most common is type 2 diabetes, usually in adults, which occurs when the body becomes resistant to insulin or doesn't make enough insulin. In the past three decades the prevalence of type 2 diabetes has risen dramatically in countries of all income levels. Type 1 diabetes, once known as juvenile diabetes or insulin-dependent diabetes, is a chronic condition in which the pancreas produces little or no insulin by itself. For people living with diabetes, access to affordable treatment, including insulin, is critical to their survival. There is a globally agreed target to halt the rise in diabetes and obesity by 2025.

About 422 million people worldwide have diabetes, the majority living in low-and middle-income countries, and 1.5 million deaths are directly attributed to diabetes each year. Both the number of cases and the prevalence of diabetes have been steadily increasing over the past few decades.

From the above World Health Organisation Report (WHO), it is clear that diabetes is dreadful disease just like cancer. Much research has been done in the development of effective blood glucose control strategies in the treatment of insulin-dependent diabetes (i.e., type 1 diabetes). Since its first proposal in the 1970s [109], *artificial pancreas* (AP) has been widely used in the blood glucose control process to compute and administrate a precise insulin dose, by using a *continuous glucose monitoring system* (CGMS) and a closed-loop controller (C. Cobelli, et al, 2011).

Tremendous progress has been made towards insulin infusion rate automation in AP using traditional control strategies such as *Proportional-Integral- Derivative* (PID), *Model Predictive Control* (MPC), and *Fuzzy Logic* (FL) (B. W. Bequette, 2005; T. Peyser, et al, 2014). A major concern is the inter- and intra- variability of the diabetic population which raises the demand for a personalized, patient specific approach of the glucose regulation.

Yasini *et al.* (2009) made an initial study on using RL to control an AP to maintain normoglycemic around 80 mg/dl. Specifically, model-free TD Q-learning algorithm was applied to compute the insulin delivery rate, without relying on an explicit model of the glucose-insulin dynamics.

Daskalaki *et al.* (2010) presented an AC controller for the estimation of insulin infusion rate *in silico* trial based on the University of Virginia/Padova type 1 diabetes simulator (B. P. Kovatchev, et al, 2009).

In an evaluation of 12-day meal scenario for 10 adults, results showed that the approach could prevent hypoglycaemia well, but hyperglycaemia could not be properly solved due to the static behaviors of the *Actor* component. The authors then proposed using daily updates of the average *basal rate* (BR) and the *insulin-to-carbohydrate* (IC) ratio in order to optimize glucose regulation (E. Daskalaki, et al, 2013), and using estimation of *information transfer* (IT) from insulin to glucose for automatic and personalized tuning of the AC approach (E. Daskalaki, et al, 2013).

Ngo *et al.* applied model-based VI method (P. D. Ngo, et al, 2018) and AC method (Ngo, P. D, et al, 2018) to reduce the fluctuation of the blood glucose in both fasting and post-meal scenarios, drawing on the Bergman's minimal insulin-glucose kinetics model (R. N. Bergman, et al, 1979) and the Hovorka model (R. Hovorka, et al, 2004) to simulate a patient.

De Paula *et al.* (2015) proposed policy learning algorithms that integrates RL with Gaussian processes to take into account glycemic variability under uncertainty, using the Ito's stochastic model of the glucose-insulin dynamics.

iii. *Anemia*

Anaemia is a condition in which the number of red blood cells or the haemoglobin concentration within them is lower than normal. Haemoglobin is needed to carry oxygen and if you have too few or abnormal red blood cells, or not enough haemoglobin, there will be a decreased capacity of the blood to carry oxygen to the body's tissues. This results in symptoms such as fatigue, weakness, dizziness and shortness of breath, among others. The optimal haemoglobin concentration needed to meet physiologic needs varies by age, sex, elevation of residence, smoking habits and pregnancy status. The most common causes of anaemia include nutritional deficiencies, particularly iron deficiency, though deficiencies in folate, vitamins B12 and A are also important causes; haemoglobinopathies; and infectious diseases, such as malaria, tuberculosis, HIV and parasitic infections.

In 2005, Gaweda *et al.* (2005) proposed treatment at the individual level in the management of renal anemia.

The FQI method was also applied by Escandell *et al.* (P2011) for discovering efficient dosing strategies based on the historical treatment data of 195 patients. An evaluation of the FQI method on a computational model that describes the effect of ESAs on the hemoglobin level showed that FQI could achieve an increment of 27.6% in the proportion of patients that are within the targeted range of hemoglobin during the period of treatment.

iv. *HIV*

The human immunodeficiency virus (HIV) targets the immune system and weakens people's defense against many infections and some types of cancer that people with healthy immune systems can fight off. As the virus destroys and impairs the function of immune cells, infected individuals gradually become immunodeficient. Immune function is typically measured by CD4 cell count. The most advanced stage of HIV infection is acquired immunodeficiency syndrome (AIDS), which can take many years to develop if not treated, depending on the individual. AIDS is defined by the development of certain cancers, infections or other severe long-term clinical manifestations.

As per report published by Who, HIV continues to be a major global public health issue, having claimed 36.3 million [27.2–47.8 million] lives so far. There is no cure for HIV infection. However, with increasing access to effective HIV prevention, diagnosis, treatment and care, including for opportunistic infections, HIV infection has become a manageable chronic health condition, enabling people living with HIV to lead long and healthy lives.

Finding effective treatment strategies for HIV-infected people is still one of the most difficult challenges in medical research. To date, the most effective method of treating HIV is to use a combination of anti-HIV drugs (antiretrovirals) in the form of Highly Active Antiretroviral Therapy (HAART) to prevent the development of drug-resistant HIV strains (B. M. Adams, et al, 2004).

Ernst et al. (2006) were the first to use RL techniques in developing Structured Treatment Interruption (STI) strategies for HIV patients.

Parbhoo (2014) applied three types of BRL methods to the problem of HIV treatment: FQI-ERT, neural FQI, and LSPI. Testing based on ten years of real clinical data from 250 HIV-infected patients at Charlotte Maxeke Johannesburg Academic Hospital in South Africa confirmed that the RL methods results were compliant with those recommended by clinicians.

The General exploration methods are unable to yield meaningful performance improvement as they can only obtain samples in the vicinity of the "non- healthy" steady state. Targeting this issue Pazis *et al.* (2013) introduced an algorithm for PAC optimal exploration in continuous state spaces.

Kawaguchi considered the time bound in a PAC exploration process (K. Kawaguchi, 2016). Results in both studies showed that the exploration algorithm could achieve far better strategies than other existing exploration strategies in HIV treatment.

B.   Mental Disorders

Mental health disorders, refers to a wide range of mental health conditions — disorders that affect your mood, thinking and behavior. Mental diseases are characterized by a long-term period of clinical treatments that usually require adaptation in the duration, dose, or type of treatment over time (S. A. Murphy, et al, 2007).

Given that the brain is a complex system and thus extremely challenging to model, applying traditional control- based methods that rely on accurate brain models in mental disease treatment is proved infeasible. Examples of mental illness include epilepsy, depression, schizophrenia, depression, anxiety disorders, and various kinds of substance addiction.

i.   *Epilepsy*

Around 1% of the world population is being affected by Epilepsy, the most common severe neurological disorders. Researchers proposed promising prediction and detection algorithms to suppress the frequency, duration and amplitude of seizures (T. N. Alotaiby, et al, 2014). However, due to lack of full understanding of seizure and its associated neural dynamics, designing optimal seizure suppression algorithms via minimal electrical stimulation has been for a long time a challenging task in treatment of epilepsy.

Guez *et al.* (2008) applied the BRL method, FQI-ERT, to optimize a deep-brain stimulation strategy for the treatment of epilepsy. En- coding the observed *Electroencephalograph* (EEG) signal as a 114-dimensional continuous feature vector, and four different simulation frequencies as the actions, the RL approach was applied to learn an optimal stimulation policy using data from an *in vitro* animal model of epilepsy (i.e., field potential recordings of seizure-like activity in slices of rat brains). Results showed that RL strategies substantially outperformed the current best stimulation strategies in the literature, reducing the incidence of seizures by 25% and total amount of electrical stimulation to the brain by a factor of about 10.

ii.   *Depression*

In this case patient suffers from dynamic mood swings. Using data from the *Sequenced Treatment Alternatives to Relieve Depression* (STAR*D) trial (A. J. Rush, et al, 2004), which is a sequenced four-stage randomized clinical trial of patients with MDD, Pineau *et al.* (2007) first applied Kernel- based BRL (D. Ormoneit and S. Sen, 2013) for constructing useful DTRs for patients with MDD. Other work tries to address the problem of nonsmooth of decision rules as well as nonregularity of the parameter estimations in traditional RL methods by proposing various extensions over default Q-learning procedure in order to increase the robustness of learning. Laber *et al.* (2014) proposed a new version of Q-learning, *interactive Q-learning* (IQ-learning), by interchanging the order of certain steps in traditional Q-learning, and showed that IQ-learning improved on Q-learning in terms of integrated mean squared error in a study of MDD.

CONCLUSION

RL presents a mathematically solid and technically sound solution to optimal decision making in various healthcare tasks challenged with noisy, multi-dimensional and incomplete data, nonlinear and complex dynamics, and particularly, sequential decision procedures with delayed evaluation feedback. This chapter focused on a state-of-the-art comprehensive survey of RL applications to a variety of decision-making problems in the area of healthcare. We have provided a summarization of the theoretical foundations and key techniques in the RL research from traditional machine learning perspective, and surveyed the broad-ranging applications of RL methods in solving problems affecting manifold areas of healthcare in Chronic diseases and Mental Disorder.

REFERENCES

Acikgoz, S. U., & Diwekar, U. M. (2010). Blood glucose regulation with stochastic optimal control for insulin-dependent diabetic patients. *Chemical Engineering Science*, *65*(3), 1227–1236. doi:10.1016/j.ces.2009.09.077

Adams, B. M., Banks, H. T., Kwon, H.-D., & Tran, H. T. (2004). Dynamic multidrug therapies for hiv: Optimal and sti control approaches. *Mathematical Biosciences and Engineering*, *1*(2), 223–241. doi:10.3934/mbe.2004.1.223 PMID:20369969

Alotaiby, T. N., Alshebeili, S. A., Alshawi, T., Ahmad, I., & El-Samie, F. E. A. (2014). Eeg seizure detection and prediction algorithms: A survey. *EURASIP Journal on Advances in Signal Processing*, *2014*(1), 183. doi:10.1186/1687-6180-2014-183

Bellman, R. E. (1983). *Mathematical methods in medicine*. World Scientific Publishing Co., Inc. doi:10.1142/0028

Bequette, B. W. (2005). A critical assessment of algorithms and challenges in the development of a closed-loop artificial pancreas. *Diabetes Technology & Therapeutics*, *7*(1), 28–47. doi:10.1089/dia.2005.7.28 PMID:15738702

Bergman, R. N., Ider, Y. Z., Bowden, C. R., & Cobelli, C. (1979). Quantitative estimation of insulin sensitivity. *American Journal of Physiology. Endocrinology and Metabolism*, *236*(6), E667. doi:10.1152/ajpendo.1979.236.6.E667 PMID:443421

Chakraborty, B., & Moodie, E. (2013). *Statistical methods for dynamic treatment regimes*. Springer. doi:10.1007/978-1-4614-7428-9

Cobelli, C., Renard, E., & Kovatchev, B. (2011). Artificial pancreas: Past, present, future. *Diabetes*, *60*(11), 2672–2682. doi:10.2337/db11-0654 PMID:22025773

Daskalaki, E. (2013). Personalized tuning of a reinforcement learning control algorithm for glucose regulation. In *2013 35th Annual International Conference of the IEEE Engineering in Medicine and Biology Society (EMBC)*. IEEE.

Daskalaki, E., Diem, P., & Mougiakakou, S. G. (2013). An actor–critic based controller for glucose regulation in type 1 diabetes. *Computer Methods and Programs in Biomedicine*, *109*(2), 116–125. doi:10.1016/j.cmpb.2012.03.002 PMID:22502983

Daskalaki, Scarnato, Diem, & Mougiakakou. (2010). *Preliminary results of a novel approach for glucose regulation using an actor-critic learning based controller.* Academic Press.

De Paula, M., Acosta, G. G., & Mart'ınez, E. C. (2015). On-line policy learning and adaptation for real-time personalization of an artificial pancreas. *Expert Systems with Applications, 42*(4), 2234–2255. doi:10.1016/j.eswa.2014.10.038

De Paula, M., Avila, L. O., & Mart, E. C. (2015). Controlling blood glucose variability under uncertainty using reinforcement learning and gaussian processes. *Applied Soft Computing, 35,* 310–332. doi:10.1016/j.asoc.2015.06.041

Dilsizian, S. E., & Siegel, E. L. (2014). Artificial intelligence in medicine and cardiac imaging: Harnessing big data and advanced computing to provide personalized medical diagnosis and treatment. *Current Cardiology Reports, 16*(1), 441. doi:10.100711886-013-0441-8 PMID:24338557

Ernst, D., Stan, G.-B., Goncalves, J., & Wehenkel, L. (2006). Clinical data based optimal sti strategies for hiv: a reinforcement learning approach. In *45th IEEE Conference on Decision and Control.* IEEE. 10.1109/CDC.2006.377527

Escandell-Montero, P., Mart'ınez-Mart'ınez, J. M., Mart'ın-Guerrero, J. D., Soria-Olivas, E., Vila-Frances, J., & Magdalena-Benedito, R. (2011). *Adaptive treatment of anemia on hemodialysis patients: A reinforcement learning approach. In CIDM2011.* IEEE.

Esteva, A., Robicquet, A., Ramsundar, B., Kuleshov, V., DePristo, M., Chou, K., Cui, C., Corrado, G., Thrun, S., & Dean, J. (2019). A guide to deep learning in healthcare. *Nature Medicine, 25*(1), 24–29. doi:10.103841591-018-0316-z PMID:30617335

Feng, M., Valdes, G., Dixit, N., & Solberg, T. D. (2018). *Machine learning in radiation oncology: Opportunities, requirements, and needs* (Vol. 8). Frontiers in Oncology.

Gaweda, A. E., Muezzinoglu, M. K., Aronoff, G. R., Jacobs, A. A., Zurada, J. M., & Brier, M. E. (2005). *Reinforcement learning approach to individualization of chronic pharmacotherapy. In IJCNN'05* (Vol. 5). IEEE.

Goldberg, Y., & Kosorok, M. R. (2012). Q-learning with censored data. *Annals of Statistics, 40*(1), 529. doi:10.1214/12-AOS968 PMID:22754029

Guez, Vincent, Avoli, & Pineau. (2008). Adaptive treatment of epilepsy via batch-mode reinforcement learning. *AAAI,* 1671–1678.

Hassani, A., & ... Reinforcement learning based control of tumor growth with chemotherapy. In *2010 International Conference on System Science and Engineering (ICSSE)*. IEEE. 10.1109/ICSSE.2010.5551776

Hovorka, R., Canonico, V., Chassin, L. J., Haueter, U., Massi-Benedetti, M., Federici, M. O., Pieber, T. R., Schaller, H. C., Schaupp, L., Vering, T., & Wilinska, M. E. (2004). Nonlinear model predictive control of glucose concentration in subjects with type 1 diabetes. *Physiological Measurement*, *25*(4), 905–920. doi:10.1088/0967-3334/25/4/010 PMID:15382830

Hu, C., Lovejoy, W. S., & Shafer, S. L. (1994). Comparison of some control strategies for three-compartment pk/pd models. *Journal of Pharmacokinetics and Biopharmaceutics*, *22*(6), 525–550. doi:10.1007/BF02353793 PMID:7473080

Humphrey. (2017). *Using reinforcement learning to personalize dosing strategies in a simulated cancer trial with high dimensional data*. Academic Press.

Jalalimanesh, A., Haghighi, H. S., Ahmadi, A., Hejazian, H., & Soltani, M. (2017). Multi-objective optimization of radiotherapy: Distributed q-learning and agent-based simulation. *Journal of Experimental & Theoretical Artificial Intelligence*, *29*(5), 1–16. doi:10.1080/0952813X.2017.1292319

Jalalimanesh, A., Haghighi, H. S., Ahmadi, A., & Soltani, M. (2017). Simulation-based optimization of radiotherapy: Agent-based modeling and reinforcement learning. *Mathematics and Computers in Simulation*, *133*, 235–248. doi:10.1016/j.matcom.2016.05.008

Jelliffe, R. W., Buell, J., Kalaba, R., Sridhar, R., & Rockwell, R. (1970). A computer program for digitalis dosage regimens. *Mathematical Biosciences*, *9*, 179–193. doi:10.1016/0025-5564(70)90103-3

Johnson, A. E., Ghassemi, M. M., Nemati, S., Niehaus, K. E., Clifton, D. A., & Clifford, G. D. (2016). Machine learning and decision support in critical care. *Proceedings of the IEEE*, *104*(2), 444–466. doi:10.1109/JPROC.2015.2501978 PMID:27765959

Kawaguchi. (2016). Bounded optimal exploration in mdp. *AAAI*, 1758–1764.

Kovatchev, Breton, Dalla Man, & Cobelli. (2009). *In silico preclinical trials: a proof of concept in closed-loop control of type 1 diabetes*. Academic Press.

Laber, E. B., Linn, K. A., & Stefanski, L. A. (2014). Interactive model building for q-learning. *Biometrika*, *101*(4), 831–847. doi:10.1093/biomet/asu043 PMID:25541562

LittmanM. L. (2015). Reinforcement learning improves behaviour from evaluative feedback. *Nature, 521*(7553), 445.

Mnih, V., Kavukcuoglu, K., Silver, D., Rusu, A. A., Veness, J., Bellemare, M. G., Graves, A., Riedmiller, M., Fidjeland, A. K., Ostrovski, G., Petersen, S., Beattie, C., Sadik, A., Antonoglou, I., King, H., Kumaran, D., Wierstra, D., Legg, S., & Hassabis, D. (2015). Human-level control through deep reinforcement learning. *Nature, 518*(7540), 529–533. doi:10.1038/nature14236 PMID:25719670

Murphy, S. A., Oslin, D. W., Rush, A. J., & Zhu, J. (2007). Methodological challenges in constructing effective treatment sequences for chronic psychiatric disorders. *Neuropsychopharmacology, 32*(2), 257–262. doi:10.1038j.npp.1301241 PMID:17091129

Ngo, P. D., Wei, S., Holubova, A., Muzik, J., & Godtliebsen, F. (2018). Reinforcement-learning optimal control for type-1 diabetes. In *2018 IEEE EMBS International Conference on Biomedical & Health Informatics (BHI)*. IEEE. 10.1109/BHI.2018.8333436

Ngo, P. D., Wei, S., Holubová, A., Muzik, J., & Godtliebsen, F. (2018). *Control of blood glucose for type-1 diabetes by using reinforcement learning with feedforward algorithm* (Vol. 2018). Computational and Mathematical Methods in Medicine.

Organization, W. H. (2005). *Preventing chronic diseases: a vital investment.* World Health Organization.

Ormoneit, D., & Sen, S. (2013). Kernel-based reinforcement learning. *Machine Learning, 49*(2-3), 161–178. PMID:23845276

Padmanabhan, R., Meskin, N., & Haddad, W. M. (2017). Reinforcement learning-based control of drug dosing for cancer chemotherapy treatment. *Mathematical Biosciences, 293*, 11–20. doi:10.1016/j.mbs.2017.08.004 PMID:28822813

Parbhoo, S. (2014). *A reinforcement learning design for HIV clinical trials* [Ph.D. dissertation].

Patel, V. L., Shortliffe, E. H., Stefanelli, M., Szolovits, P., Berthold, M. R., Bellazzi, R., & Abu-Hanna, A. (2009). The coming of age of artificial intelligence in medicine. *Artificial Intelligence in Medicine, 46*(1), 5–17. doi:10.1016/j.artmed.2008.07.017 PMID:18790621

Pazis & Parr. (2013). Pac optimal exploration in continuous space Markov decision processes. *AAAI*.

Peyser, T., Dassau, E., Breton, M., & Skyler, J. S. (2014). The artificial pancreas: Current status and future prospects in the management of diabetes. *Annals of the New York Academy of Sciences*, *1311*(1), 102–123. doi:10.1111/nyas.12431 PMID:24725149

Pineau, J., Bellemare, M. G., Rush, A. J., Ghizaru, A., & Murphy, S. A. (2007). Constructing evidence-based treatment strategies using methods from computer science. *Drug and Alcohol Dependence*, *88*, S52–S60. doi:10.1016/j.drugalcdep.2007.01.005 PMID:17320311

Pineau, J., Guez, A., Vincent, R., Panuccio, G., & Avoli, M. (2009). Treating epilepsy via adaptive neurostimulation: A reinforcement learning approach. *International Journal of Neural Systems*, *19*(04), 227–240. doi:10.1142/S0129065709001987 PMID:19731397

Rush, A. J., Fava, M., Wisniewski, S. R., Lavori, P. W., Trivedi, M. H., Sackeim, H. A., Thase, M. E., Nierenberg, A. A., Quitkin, F. M., Kashner, T. M., Kupfer, D. J., Rosenbaum, J. F., Alpert, J., Stewart, J. W., McGrath, P. J., Biggs, M. M., Shores-Wilson, K., Lebowitz, B. D., Ritz, L., & Niederehe, G.the STAR*D Investigators Group. (2004). Sequenced treatment alternatives to relieve depression (star* d): Rationale and design. *Controlled Clinical Trials*, *25*(1), 119–142. doi:10.1016/S0197-2456(03)00112-0 PMID:15061154

Schaefer, A. J., Bailey, M. D., Shechter, S. M., & Roberts, M. S. (2005). *Modeling medical treatment using markov decision processes. In Operations Research and Health Care*. Springer.

Soliman, Y. M. (2014). *Personalized medical treatments using novel reinforcement learning algorithms*. arXiv preprint arXiv:1406.3922

Yasini, S., Naghibi Sistani, M. B., & Karimpour, A. (2009). Agent-based simulation for blood glucose. *International Journal of Applied Science, Engineering and Technology*, *5*, 89–95.

Zhao, Y., Kosorok, M. R., & Zeng, D. (2009). Reinforcement learning design for cancer clinical trials. *Statistics in Medicine*, *28*(26), 3294–3315. doi:10.1002im.3720 PMID:19750510

Chapter 9

Artificial Intelligence:
A Tool for Detection of Pandemics

Kumud Pant
Graphic Era University (Deemed), India

Bhasker Pant
Graphic Era University (Deemed), India

Somya Sinha
Graphic Era University (Deemed), India

ABSTRACT

The spread of the COVID-19 pandemic made us rethink the need for integrating modern scientific algorithms in decision support as well as medical systems. This chapter focuses on the on-going efforts throughout the world for tackling the COVID-19 pandemic with the use of artificial intelligence and machine learning algorithms. The chapter also compiles the various efforts made internationally for providing solution to this disease. The examples of use of algorithms like artificial neural network, fuzzy clustering, and support vector machines for both the disease recognition as well as in medical aid have been stated. Finally, the chapter also reiterates the need for developing even more advanced algorithms and prediction systems in case of future pandemic outbreaks due to ever mutating microorganisms and other lifestyle problems. More than just scientific and governmental endeavors, prudent handling of any emergency health situation requires awareness as well as self-discipline exercised by inhabitants of any country.

INTRODUCTION

The unexpected, unprecedented global fire of COVID-19 pandemic is the best explanation for practically experiencing a pandemic at large. While a pandemic

DOI: 10.4018/978-1-6684-6646-9.ch009

breaks all the boundaries of nations on the globe, epidemic is the spread of a disease within a particular localized geographical area (Centre for Disease Control, 2012). Yellow fever and small pox are few examples. The third category is endemic where the disease outbreak is confined to a particular geographical location but is consistent in its presence. The best example is malaria endemically found in tropical African nations as well as central and South America (Columbia Mailman School of Public Health, 2022). Few other significant pandemics from yesteryears are summarized in Table 1 (Columbia Mailman School of Public Health, 2022; Piret & Boivin, 2021).

Table 1. Major pandemic outbreaks of the world

S. No.	Details of the Epidemics/ Pandemics	Causative Organism	Duration of the Most Severe Effect	Time Period in Years
1.	The black death (Bubonic Plague)	Yersinia pestis	Four (4) years	1346-1353
2.	American Plague, Small Pox	Small pox virus		16th Century
3.	1st Cholera Pandemic (CP) 2nd CP 3rd CP 4th CP 5th CP 6th CP 7th CP	Vibrio cholera	Seven (7) years Eight (8) years Seventeen (17) years Twelve (12) years Five (5) years Twenty four (24) years Ongoing	1817-1824 1827-1835 1839-1856 1863-1875 1881-1886 1899-1923 1961- Currently Ongoing
4.	The Russian Flu	Influenza virus Influenza A/H3N8	One (1) year	1889-1893
5.	The Spanish Flu	Influenza virus Influenza A/H1N1	Two (2) years	1918-1920
6.	The Asian Flu	Various Avian Flu Viruses specially Influenza virus Influenza A/H2N2	One (1) year	1957-1959
7.	The Hong Long Flu	Influenza virus Influenza A/H3N2	Two (2) years	1968-1970
8.	AIDS	HUMAN Immunodeficiency Virus (HIV)	Still going on	1981-Currently ongoing
9.	Severe Acute Respiratory Syndrome	SARS-CoV	One (1) year	2002-2003
10.	Swine flu	Influenza virus Influenza A/H1N1	ONE (1) YEAR	2009-2010
11.	Middle East Respiratory Syndrome	MERS Virus	Ongoing	2015- Currently Ongoing
12.	COVID-19	SARS-CoV-2	Ongoing	2019-Currently Ongoing

Artificial Intelligence

What Is Artificial Intelligence?

Artificial intelligence (AI) is the intelligence of the machine which is the result of human intervention and training into making a machine intelligent enough to perform tasks as desired by humans. It is actually 'Human made Intelligence', similar to 'Human made Organs' or 'Artificial Organs'. One of the subsets of AI is Machine Learning (ML). The machine learning field deals with using various computer algorithms for making predictions or decisions without the need for programming the system. The ML algorithms help the computers or machines learn from the data having once trained the system, without the need to do it again and again (KNN at Javapoint, 2022). The most popular machine learning algorithms are shown in figure 1.

Algorithms in AI Used for Disease Diagnosis

K-Nearest Neighbor (KNN) Algorithm (KNN at Javapoint, 2022)

General Introduction

1. It is a type of supervised learning algorithm and one of the simplest one.
2. It learns from the available case data and assigns the new data into the group or class to which it is most similar.
3. It stores the entire available data and after calculating the similarity classifies a new data point into it.
4. Can be used for both regression and classification analyses but majorly used for classification.
5. It is a non-parametric as well as lazy algorithm i.e. it makes no assumptions on data to be analyzed as well does not trains from dataset. Instead performs the required action at the time of classification. It calculates the Euclidean distance of K number of neighbors.

Naïve Bayes (NB) algorithm (Naïve Bayes at Javapoint, 2022).

General Introduction

1. It is also a supervised learning classification algorithm. Made of two words i.e. Naive and Bayes. Naïve word is used in nomenclature to signify the fact

that presence of a particular attribute is not dependent on the presence of other, moreover each attribute makes and equal contribution to the final outcome.

2. NB are actually ensemble classification algorithms with basic idea derived from Bayes Theorem.
3. The theorem is based on determining probability of occurrence of an event based on probability of the prior.
4. The equation for algorithm is $P(A / B) = \dfrac{P(B / A)P(A)}{P(B)}$, where P(A/B) is posterior probability and P(B/A) is the likelihoodprobability.**P(A)** is the prior probability and **P(B)** is the marginal probability.

Support Vector Machine (SVM at Javapoint, 2022)

General Introduction

1. It is one of the most popular classification and regression analysis algorithms. It works by unraveling the confines or boundary between data points in the dataset based on the attributes of the data. This decision boundary line is termed as hyperplane.
2. For construction of the hyperplane the data points or the support vectors are chosen in such a way that margins of the classifier is maximized. These data points are actually the extreme points or points nearest to the hyperplane that help in construction of the hyperplane, called as support vectors, therefore the name Support Vector Machine (SVM) (SVM at Javapoint, 2022).
3. SVM algorithms can be divided into two categories based on type of data points in dataset. They are Linear and Non-linear SVM.
4. For data separable into two classes with the use of a straight line Linear SVM is used and classifier is termed as linear classifier. It uses two dimensions only viz. 'x' and 'y', since data points can be easily separated in a 2-D space with the use of a single line. Out of the many lines or hyperplanes possible, to segregate the data in a 2-D space, the one with maximum margin on both the sides is chosen. This maximum margin hyperplane is termed as optimal hyperplane. The SVM algorithm is built with the same intention to broaden the margin (SVM at Javapoint, 2022).
5. For a non-linear data (where data points follow random order in contrary to sequential in linear data), single line for partitioning data is not possible. The need for separating the data therefore demands introduction of another or third dimension 'z'.
6. SVM uses an ensemble mathematical function called as kernel functions to transform the data into required format. It is a measure of similarity between

points in the dataset. The kernel functions help in increasing the dimension and forming the hyperplane for data classification in higher dimension (SVM at geeksforgeeks, 2022; SVM Kernel Function at techvidan, 2022). The number of dimensions can be infinitely increased with the use of kernels.

7. The most popular kernel functions are Linear kernel, Radial Basis Kernel (RBF kernel), Polynomial Kernel

Principle Component Analysis (PCA) (PCA at Javapoint, 2022)

General Introduction

1. It is a common unsupervised machine learning algorithm and feature extraction protocol used for dimensionality reduction of dataset using statistical techniques. The concepts of variance and covariance and Eigen values and Eigen factors are used in PCA.
2. The reduced number of features or transformed features or the most significant features in the dataset is obtained through orthogonal transformation of correlated features into set of linearly uncorrelated features (PCA at javapoint, 2022). These features are termed as Principle Components (PCs).
3. PCs are the most representative features of the class of a dataset. The transformed dataset has smaller number of features with retention of maximum information in the original dataset.
4. The various steps of PCA are (PCA at Javapoint, 2022; Avijeet, 2022).
   a. Data normalization-
   b. Covariance matrix construction
   c. Finding the Eigen Vectors and Eigen Values
   d. Arrangement of Eigen vectors in decreasing order and selection of PCs.
   e. Removal of less important or unimportant features.
5. PCA so far has been used in dimensionality reduction in various AI applications like healthcare data analysis, image analysis, stick exchange data analysis, finding hidden patterns in data with high dimensions (PCA at Javapoint, 2022; Avijeet, 2022).

Random forest algorithms (Random Forest at Javapoint, 2022; Random Forest at Analyticsvidhya, 2021)

General Introduction

1. This algorithm again falls under the category of supervised learning technique and can be used for both classification and regression. It utilizes the concept

of ensemble learning that incorporates more than one classifier for improving the classification accuracy. Based on multiple decision trees built on subsets of the dataset and majority votes, the final predictions or output is presented. To do away with the problem of data overfitting more number of trees are preferred.

Clustering algorithms (Clustering at Geeksforgeek, 2022; Clustering at Javapoint, 2022)

One of the unsupervised learning technique is clustering. The meaning is very much apparent with the fact that no labeling or categorization of the dataset is done or no supervision of the data is done. In this technique the uncategorized or unlabeled data is clustered or grouped on the basis of similarity in data points. The similarity in data points can be in the form of shape, size, color and many more. Each cluster or group is then assigned a unique identity. Clustering is observed in daily life also, example is clustering of similar things together in a departmental store. The main clustering methods are Partitioning Clustering, Density based Clustering, Distribution model based Clustering, Hierarchical Clustering, Fuzzy Clustering.

Partitioning Clustering

It is a centroid based method where distance between data points in a cluster is least in comparison to centroid in other clusters. Example is K-means clustering.

Density-Based Clustering

The densest areas are connected to form clusters. The shape of the distribution is arbitrary and it is the sparse area that partitions the cluster or the dense areas.

Distribution Model-Based Clustering

The clustering is based on Gaussian Distribution. The example is Expectation-Maximization clustering that uses Gaussian Mixture Model (GMM).

Hierarchical Clustering

The number of clusters are not required to be pre fixed therefore this technique is a different approach to partition clustering. Example is Agglomerative Hierarchical algorithm.

Fuzzy Clustering

This clustering based approach falls under soft clustering method where the data point may belong to multiple clusters or groups example of this clustering approach is Fuzzy C-means algorithm.

Dimensionality Reduction Algorithm

The Curse of Dimensionality

The increase in dimension or attributes in a dataset may not always be helpful in increasing the accuracy of the classifier. Rather the attributes may show redundancy hence leading to overfitting and also increase in complexity of the classifier. Therefore, it is necessary to eliminate attributes with redundancy as well as choose the attribute(s) or features that represent the class best. Therefore, many algorithms are developed to reduce the dimension of the dataset or converting dataset with higher dimension or more number of attributes to lower dimension with lesser number of attributes, without compromising the accuracy and predictive capabilities of the classifier. The prominent ones are listed.

a.   Principle Component Analysis (PCA)
b.   Backward Elimination
c.   Forward Selection
d.   Score Comparison
e.   Missing Value Ratio
f.   Low Variance Filter
g.   High Correlation Filter
h.   Random Forest
i.   Factor Analysis
j.   Auto Encoder

Correlation and Regression Algorithms (Regression at javapoint, 2022; Statistical Language at Australian Bureau of Statistics, 2022)

Regression is the analysis to understand the association between dependent and independent variables. In other words, it helps to understand how the dependent variable changes with independent variable. To depict this dependency or relationship a graph is plotted between the variables. With the help of this plot machine learning algorithm based models are then used to make predictions about the data. The various kinds of regression analysis are Linear Regression, Polynomial Regression, Support

Vector Regression, Decision Tree Regression, Random Forest Regression, Ridge Regression, Lasso Regression, Logistic Regression

Correlation in statistics represents strength between variables or relationship between variables. The correlation is said to be found if change in the value of one variable observes change in the value of the other variable too. The correlation is depicted by symbol 'r', that represents relationship between variables. The relationship between variables can exist be of three types.

1. Positive Correlation
   When both the variables increase or decrease together it is called as positive correlation.
2. Negative Correlation
   When variables show opposite trend of increase in one and decrease in the other it is called as negative correlation.
3. Zero Correlation

The absence of linear relationship is depicted by zero correlation. In simple words one variable may increase or decrease while the other may remain constant

USE OF ARTIFICIAL INTELLIGENCE (AI) IN PANDEMIC DETECTION

March, 2020 saw the declaration of COVID-19 as a pandemic by the World Health Organization (WHO), a specialized agency of United Nations taking care of health of all humans of this world (WHO Constitution, 2020; Anjan, 2021). There are 632,533,408 cases worldwide and 2,104,828 new reported cases in last 7 days, according to WHO Coronavirus (COVID-19) Dashboard, till 16th November, 2022 and retrieved on the same date (WHO Coronavirus Dashboard, 2022). Since the time it was first reported till today Corona virus transcended all boundaries, all regions and all age groups to have caused irreparable damage to human lives. Moreover with various mutants of the virus constantly evolving and spread throughout the world, it posed a challenge to the intelligentsia for developing systems for not only early detection virus but also predicting upcoming mutants and their lethality.

The best use of AI has been seen during recent times of COVID pandemic. Although few examples of use of AI algorithms have been seen in the past but the best implementation has been observed for detection as well as prediction of spread of Corona virus. The major studies are compiled further in the chapter.

The applications of Artificial Intelligence algorithms can be further trifurcated into classes viz.

Figure 1. Various machine learning algorithms used in artificial intelligence

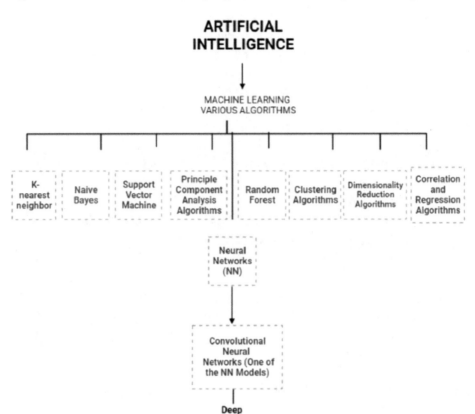

1. Recognizing and detecting infected individuals.
2. Providing assistance to health workers through disease diagnosis and also offering help in formulating effective treatment.
3. Monitor and predict epidemic spread.

Recognizing and Detecting Infected Individuals

Majority of the disease spread can be averted if the individuals containing the pathogen can be identified at the early stages. This is majorly true for all infectious diseases including COVID-19. Following the same protocol majority countries started deploying temperature check facility at airports. Thermal cameras were used to pin point individuals with more than the normal body temperature. In the period prior to COVD-19 also multiple steps were taken to identify and recognize individuals with high chance of influenza, with the use of Artificial Neural Network (ANN) and

Fuzzy Clustering algorithms (Sun, 2015). The classifier predictor was trained using attributes like respiration, body temperature and heart-beat. The clustering algorithm of fuzzy was used since it can help in reaching the most appropriate decision based on combination of belongingness of various data points in a particular cluster. This algorithm is different from hard clustering since data points can belong to all clusters but with varying membership values ranging from 0 to 1. Therefore, is suitable in diagnosis of a trend in bigger population.

COVID-19 is not the only pandemic to have hit us as can be seen through the historical account of major pandemics given in table 1, nor it is the last. What we need actually is modern technology like artificial intelligence (AI) based tools for predicting, screening and detecting the onset and also the seriousness of the spread before it actually happens. The development of such tools can help in controlling as well as mitigating the effect to a large extent.

One such AI based model developed by J. Laguarta et al., could predict with an accuracy of almost 99%, person's suffering from COVID-19 just from patterns of phone recorded coughs (Laguarta, 2020). The differentiating patterns were recognized with the help of just four indications specific to COVID-19 patients' viz. vocal cord strength, sentiment, lung and respiratory performance, and muscular degradation. This study demonstrated the use of machine learning algorithm of Neural Network called as ResNet50 for achieving this feat.

An excellent review of cough sound analysis with the help algorithms of artificial intelligence is given by Kawther S. Alqudaihi et al. (Alqudaihi, 2021). This review highlights the fact that use of artificial intelligence has been used previously also for detection of cough based diseases.

The use of wearable devices for crowdsensing model development have also been researched and advocated by many scientific groups. A machine learning based model developed by Harsh Mankodiya et al., using Support Vector Machines (SVM) was used along with a wearable device for detection of individuals with COVID-19, in crowded spaces. The device could also inform about the geographical coordinates of the person wearing it along with use of YOLOv5 object detection method for real time tracking of the individual on CCTV (Mankodiya, 2022). Similarly, Nguyen et al. worked on development of wearable face mask fitted with biosensors for detecting presence of the virus in 90 minutes in the individual wearing it (Nguyen, 2021).

Not only detection of symptoms and hence the person exhibiting the symptoms is important but also the fact that preliminary measures like social distancing, if followed properly, can avoid spread of pandemics on a bigger level. Deep learning, which is an offshoot of artificial intelligence can be used for object detection, and therefore can be envisioned for its application in designing strategies against spread of pandemic. Deep learning is based on artificial neural network (ANN) and uses Convolutional Neural Network (CNN) based object detection. Deep learning based models like YOLO (You Only Look Once), single-shot detector (SSD), and R-CNN are also being used for object detection. In a model proposed by Erbahiim et al., deep learning has been used for individual detection with subtraction of the background (Kajabad, 2019). A model to detect static crowds has also been developed using SVM. The SVM is trained to locate presence of spots, indicating group of people. The groups are later extracted using text features (Manfredi, 2014). A. Alahi et al., in 2014 (before the COVID pandemic) suggested use of real time pedestrians detection (Alahi, 2014). Similar monitoring systems have been proposed for smart cities (Kaur, 2018; Tomar, 2018). Sangeeta Yadav e al., in the similar lines, proposed a novel real-time crowd monitoring and management system for social distance classification. The group employed YOLO v4 object detection model to separate people from background and further the detected people were tracked by bounding boxes using Deepsort technique (Yadav, 2022).

A detailed review on development of contactless personal identification system with the application of artificial intelligence algorithms has been given by Shinpei Matsuda et al. (Matsuda, 2022).

All the systems discussed above can be helpful in understanding the follow-up of norms of public safety by common people as well as in developing protocols for detection of upcoming pandemics using various attributes of the pathogen.

Providing assistance to health workers through disease diagnosis and also offering help in formulating effective treatment

The timely and early diagnosis of any disease ensures the formulation of effective therapeutic regime and offers aid in combating it as well as mitigating the pathogen spread. Many scientific endeavors are used for disease diagnosis as well as detection.

During the COVID times, Reverse transcription polymerase chain reaction (RT-PCR), was the most used for diagnosis. As study was done on results obtained using RT-PCR test, many false negative results were also obtained (Arevalo-Rodriguez, 2020). Moreover, the delay in results also was a bottleneck to have halted actual medical prescription (Pecoraro, 2022). According to Fu JYL et al. (Fu, 2021), the newer strains of virus may not be detected through this technique. Therefore, other techniques should also be used along with RT-PCR with the use of AI algorithms to diagnose disease with better accuracy and precision.

Techniques like CT scans, chest X-rays, various disease markers, MRI, Ultrasound, audio analysis and Rapid Antigen Test (RAT) can also be used alone or in combination, with the application of machine learning antigens to enhance diagnostic powers of laboratory techniques.

The use of various AI algorithms along with integration of multiple techniques to enhance quality of COVID patient detection is given in table 2.

Other laboratory techniques like CT scan and X-ray images can also be used for disease detection. CT scan creates 3D images and 360 degree view of the body

Table 2. Diagnosis using AI algorithms and RTPCR

Authors	AI Algorithm Used	Name of the Model Developed	Accuracy	Sensitivity	Specificity	AUC	F1 Score
EmreÖzbilge et al. (Ozbulge, 2022)	Deep convolutional neural network (DCNN)	MobileNetV2 model	1	1	1	1	1
Alouani et al. (Alouani, 2021)	DCNN without threshold cycle (C_t) value	qPCRdeepNet	TP= 146 FP=0 TN=3882 FN=2				
Lee et al. (Lee, 2022)	Long Short Term Memory Neural Network (LSTM)			90.00%	92.54%	91.27%	

part under examination, therefore has more detailed view of the problem. When coupled with AI classifiers the detection only takes few seconds for abnormalities to be located. However, the use of computational algorithms with CT scan requires knowledge of both image processing as well as deep learning. In the initial step of the classifier region of interest (ROI) is located, the rest of the tissues not falling in the ROI are removed in the second step and by using the deep learning models classification is performed as the final step (Khanna, 2022). The AI algorithms used with CT scan are summarized below. The noteworthy efforts made post COVID era especially in 2021 and 2022 are considered for further description.

Carvalho et al. used an amalgamation of CNN and multilayer perceptron along with VGG16, VGG19, ResNet50 to train and test models of CT scanned COVID patients (Carvalho, 2021). The use of deep neural network (DNN) along with CNN was done by Mukherjee et al. They combined X-ray dataset along with CT scan and obtained an accuracy of 96.28% for the classifier (Mukherjee, 2021).

Shalbaf et al. made use of various CNN like InceptionV3, NasNet, ResNet50, SeResnet50, Xception, DenseNet121 for the analysis. the authors used images from COVID-19 and normal individuals. The accuracy was found to be 85% for the classification (Shalabaf, 2021). For extending the usability of AI algorithms MobileNet has also been used for COVID detection. Since MobileNet CNN architecture is smaller and a faster one therefore its portability can be increased in the form of mobile apps. The same has been used by Nayak et al. along with other CNN architectures like VGG-16, ResNet-50 etc. for disease diagnosis using X-ray images (Nayak, 2021).

X-ray imaging for diagnosis was heavily used during COVID times for disease detection and diagnosis. However, it has limitations that other cough related disorders like pneumonia, tuberculosis etc. are difficult to distinguish from corona born cough infections. Therefore, potentiating the analysis through X-ray images,requires usage of other advance techniques and algorithms. Notable efforts have been made in this direction by incorporating AI algorithms for X-ray image analysis.

Convolutional neural network (CNN) is network architecture for deep learning. It was used by Panwar et al. with the name 'nCOVnet' for identifying image features of healthy and infected individuals with accuracy of 97% for true positives (Panwar, 2020). Another models COVIDX-Net was developed using VGG19 convolutional neural network along with Google MobileNet, the model could classify the images with an accuracy of 90% (Hemdan, 2020). Narin et al. in 2021 used the ResNet (50, 101 and 152) in CNN along with InceptionV3 and V2 (Narin, 2021). The advantage of this model lay in the fact that COVID patients, healthy patients as well as pneumonic patients could be distinguished with high accuracy.

Prediction of severity of the disease is another strategic planning for tackling any pandemic situation. This can help in designing and devising better therapeutic agents as well as patient care protocols. AI algorithms have been used to predict the severity of CORONA along with output from clinical techniques like X-ray images. A VGG16 architecture based classifier was developed for severity prediction using chest X-ray images by Heidari et al. This transfer learning method gave accuracy of 98% (Heidari, 2020). A DenseNet CNN architecture based model was used by Cohen et al. to predict ct the severity of the disease (Joseph Paul Cohen, 2020).

Through various computational algorithms, clinical markers of a disease have been analyzed to make useful observations that could further aid the healthcare workers as well scientists in designingdisease related prognosis. LASSO regression analysis algorithm used by Li et al., on unique disease variables, led to the conclusion that blood group A patients were could meet more fatal consequences in comparison to other blood groups. The same study also concluded that with decrease in temperature disease transmission of corona virus spreads faster (Li, 2020). Through the use of conventional machine learning algorithms like random forest, study of haematological markers along with RT-PCR could predict presence of COVID-19 with 81% accuracy (Tschoellitsch, 2021).

Similarly, AI algorithms have also been used with magnetic resonance imaging (MRI) and ultrasound results as well for disease diagnosis with greater precision (Jaime Gil-Rodriguez, 2022).

Finding Effective Drug Molecule, Developing Vaccine and Designing Treatment Using AI

In the quest for unraveling new molecules with anti-viral activity use of artificial intelligence in super computers cannot be overlooked (Joseph, 2020). Deep learning algorithms have also been developed for prediction of properties of various molecules as well as creation of new molecules with desired effects (Zhong, 2020). In another good study, artificial intelligence was extended to docking interaction in the form of deep docking model to predict the docking scores for number of compounds along with screening of molecules with therapeutic potential in less time. Moreover, the disbursement of the data for the public opens up the possibility of further research as well as drug design for more diseases and pandemics (Arshadi, 2020). ML algorithms have been implemented for viral therapies including drug repurposing as well as for prediction of inhibitors (Ge, 2021). Drug repurposing has recently been a topic of intense research and discussion where already approved old drugs are implicated for treating new diseases. Here also AI algorithms have been applied successfully, more specifically for COVID-19 (Arshadi, 2020). Li et al proposed 30 drugs as repurposable for COVID-19 using genomic sequences molecular network study with implementation of artificial intelligence algorithms (Li Xu, 2021).

The challenge with any pandemic lies in the fact that it does not give enough time to prepare and test new things as deterrent against it. Due to limited time, the possibility of trial and error does not exist and combat has to be designed at the fastest of the pace. Vaccine development for corona virus similarly faced safety concerns as well as issues of complete effectiveness (Rawat, 2021). AI has been used for better understanding of proteins of the pathogen with unraveling of cryptic and novel dug targets. Targets were predicted from corona virus with Vaxign machine learning based reverse vaccinology approach for bringing to fore novel vaccine candidates (Ong, 2020).

In a work with the similar potency RNN (recurrent neural network) has been used to understand and predict targets for vaccine development (Crossman, 2020). A ML-based programs namely OptiAX has been developed for development of peptide vaccines and the other program called EvalMax has been developed by analyzing genetic composition of various ethnic populations and the haplotype frequencies of human leukocyte antigens (HLA) that can work with peptides that provide even heightened immune response. Both the programs have been developed by researchers at MIT computer science center and AI lab (Liu Ge, 2021; Liu, Ge, 2020).

Monitor and Predict Epidemic Spread

The use of AI algorithms has been seen not only for formulating effective treatment but also to monitor as well as make predictions about spread of the disease. A noteworthy technology is BlueDot (https://bluedot.global/). It is a Canadian software company headquartered in Toronto, Canada. Established in 2013 it initially was motivated by SARS outbreak in 2004. Whereas during COVID-19 pandemic first time on January 5th, 2019 BlueDot sent a warning to its users six days prior about the impending danger in China, that later caused havoc in the world in the form of COVID-19 (CNB News, 2022; MIT Technology Review, 2021; Bilal, 2021; Stieg, 2020).

The use of AI and MLTs has been seen in BlueDot technology along with natural language processing algorithms (NLP) to decipher contents from more than 10,000 official and media sources from more than 60 languages. The technology also collected data from various sources including airline ticketing data. After combining data from all the resources and training with the data of computer algorithms, hot spots and cold spots of infection were identified. The company then used this prediction as a warning system for its clients located in these areas about disease severity and spread (Martins, 2019; BlueDot, 2022).

Metabiota (https://www.metabiota.com/), is another venture that uses artificial intelligence and big data analytics. With inputs from flight data it could very well in advance predict the corona virus outbreak in countries like Japan, Thailand, Taiwan etc. days before cases were observed in these countries (Heilweil, 2020; Allam, 2020).

MetaBiota headquartered at San Francisco combines power of AI, MLTs, Big Data and Neuro Linguistic Programming algorithms (NLP). It defers from BlueDot in its use of data from social media also. Since the main clients of Metabiota are insurance companies therefore it has been of help in making decisions with minimum risks. The information generated by Metabiota can also be prudently used by other government and non-government agencies in decision making during any disease outbreak.

INDIA AND ARTIFICIAL INTELLIGENCE IN TACKLING COVID-19 PANDEMIC

The world health organization's (WHO) recommended doctor patient ratio is 1:1000 while India has ratio of 1:1456 (according to economic survey of India, 2019-20) (How India Fights COVID with AI at analyticsindiamag, 2021). Moreover, the use of artificial intelligence in healthcare sector is just 1.9% (How India Fights COVID with AI at analyticsindiamag, 2021). Hence, the need is felt for more inclusive role to be played by technology in health system. Few notable mentions are use of AI assisted technology to capture those who don't wear or misuse masks. This has been possible with the help of images captures by CCTV installed at crowded public places. In a similar example Glimpse Analytics of Pune, Maharashtra has used AI as an alert system to warn commercial outlets and offices of violation in COVID norms during pandemic period. At multiple centers throughout India CT scans and X-rays have been analyzed with integrated technology using AI and machine learning algorithms for more accurate disease analysis. India's premiere government agency namely Defence Research and Development Organisation (DRDO) has developed AI enabled intelligent COVID detection application software ATMAN AI. The software has been used for distinguishing COVID-19 images from rest of the chest images with other diseases. ATMAN AI employs Deep Convolutional Neural Network for proper image classification. Moreover, it has been made portable for use by integrating into mobiles, tablets etc. The system showed accuracy of almost 97% on data of chest X-rays. Another technology for diagnosis named as COVIRAP was initiated by IIT Kharagpur. This tool has multiple components like control unit, detection unit for analysis of genome and smart phone application to display findings from the system.

Both Accenture and Microsoft collaborated with Indian Government's digital India Corporation and came up with an intuitive chatbot named MyGov Saathi, built on artificial intelligence that provided citizens with updated information on COVID-19. The chatbot could provide services to approximately 50,000 users on daily basis. It again worked on NLP and AI platforms.

WhatsApp is free messenger application for smart phones that makes use of internet to send messages, images and also audio video files. Due to its less cost and accessibility the app is highly popular and is used by more than 390 million users in India. Realizing the immense potential in communicating with Indians a WhatsApp based introbot was developed. The introbot was of great help during COVID times since it made available for users database of beds, oxygen cylinders, and other essential medical things. It is an AI-community manager that helped people in more than 300 Indian cities.

In another initiative a conversational AI platform Yellow Messenger launched Yellow Messenger Cares. The Messenger was developed with an aim to provide assistance though chatbots for hospitals, NGO's etc.

The AI and MLTs are being rapidly used in drug repurposing also. A joint Indo-German venture 'Innoplexus' is working on repurposing Hydroxychloroquine (anti-malarial drug) and Remdesivir (Anti Ebola drug) for COVID-19 (How are AI-based solutions being used to combat COVID-19? at indiaa.gov.in).

There are many more examples from India and Indian subcontinent where use of AI and MLTs was evident during COVID-19 pandemic but future preparedness is required to further control spread of pandemic in future.

CONCLUSION

The use of artificial algorithms has been tremendously observed in devising novel therapies as well as detection and also prediction of spread with special context to COVID-19. The future of pandemic cannot be seen but preparedness can always be done for any unforeseen event, since humanity is at a greater risk. This has been seen in recent COVID-19 outbreak where worldwide millions of people lost their lives and livelihood. Therefore, envisaging any future outbreak due to rapidly mutating microorganism, calls for development of even advance algorithms for predicting any future calamity.

REFERENCES

Alahi, A., Bierlaire, M., & Vandergheynst, P. (2014). Robust realtimepedestrians detection in urban environments with lowresolution cameras. *Transportation Research Part C, Emerging Technologies*, *39*, 113–128. doi:10.1016/j.trc.2013.11.019

Allam, Z., Dey, G., & Jones, D. S. (2020). Artificial intelligence (AI) provided early detection of the coronavirus (COVID-19) in China and will influence future urban health policy internationally. *AI, 1*(2), 156–165. . doi:10.3390/ai1020009

Alouani, D. J., Rajapaksha, R. R. P., Jani, M., Rhoads, D. D., & Sadri, N. (2021). Specificity of SARS-CoV-2 real-time PCR improved by deep learning analysis. *Journal of Clinical Microbiology*, *59*(6), e02959–e20. doi:10.1128/JCM.02959-20 PMID:33731417

Alqudaihi, K. S., Aslam, N., Khan, I. U., Almuhaideb, A. M. A. M., Alsunaidi, S. J., Ibrahim, N. M. A. R., Alhaidari, F. A., Shaikh, F. S., Alsenbel, Y. M., Alalharith, D. M., Alharthi, H. M., Alghamdi, W. M., & Alshahrani, M. S. (2021, July 15). Cough sound detection and diagnosis using artificial intelligence techniques: Challenges and opportunities. *IEEE Access : Practical Innovations, Open Solutions*, *9*, 102327–102344. doi:10.1109/ACCESS.2021.3097559 PMID:34786317

Arevalo-Rodriguez, I., Buitrago-Garcia, D., Simancas-Racines, D., Zambrano-Achig, P., Del Campo, R., Ciapponi, A., Sued, O., Martinez-García, L., Rutjes, A. W., Low, N., Bossuyt, P. M., Perez-Molina, J. A., & Zamora, J. (2020, December 10). False-negative results of initial RT-PCR assays for COVID-19: A systematic review. *PLoS One*, *15*(12), e0242958. doi:10.1371/journal.pone.0242958 PMID:33301459

Avijeet, B. (2022, November 30). *PCA in machine learning – Your complete guide to principal component analysis*. https://www.simplilearn.com/tutorials/machine-learning-tutorial/principal-component-analysis

Bilal, M. (2021). *Digital health: Opportunities for entrepreneurs, scientists and doctors*. https://propakistani.pk/2021/06/23/digital-health-opportunities-for-entrepreneurs-scientists-and-doctors/

BlueDot. (n.d.). *Better public health surveillance for infectious diseases.* https:// bluedot.global/products/explorer/

Bullock, J., Luccioni, A., Hoffman Pham, K., Sin Nga Lam, C., & Luengo-Oroz, M. (2020). Mapping the landscape of artificial intelligence applications against COVID-19. *Journal of Artificial Intelligence Research, 69,* 807–845. doi:10.1613/ jair.1.12162

Carvalho, E. D., Silva, R. R. V., Araújo, F. H. D., Rabelo, R. A. L., & de Carvalho Filho, A. O. (2021, September). An approach to the classification of COVID-19 based on CT scans using convolutional features and genetic algorithms. *Computers in Biology and Medicine, 136,* 104744. doi:10.1016/j.compbiomed.2021.104744 PMID:34388465

Clustering in machine learning. (n.d.a). https://www.geeksforgeeks.org/clustering-in-machine-learning/

Clustering in machine learning. (n.d.b). https://www.javatpoint.com/clustering-in-machine-learning

Cohen, J. P., Dao, L., Roth, K., Morrison, P., Bengio, Y., Abbasi, A. F., Shen, B., Mahsa, H. K., Ghassemi, M., Li, H., & Duong, T. Q. (2020, July). Predicting COVID-19 pneumonia severity on chest X-ray with deep learning. *Cureus, 12*(7), e9448. doi:10.7759/cureus.9448 PMID:32864270

CrossmanL. (2020).04.20.046920. Leverging Deep Learning to stimulate coronavirus Spike proteins has the potential to predict future Zoonotic sequences. bioRxiv, 2020. https://doi.org/ doi:10.1101/2020.04.20.046920

Fu, J. Y. L., Chong, Y. M., Sam, I. C., & Chan, Y. F. (2022). SARS-CoV-2 multiplex RT-PCR to detect variants of concern (VOCs) in Malaysia, between January to May 2021. *Journal of Virological Methods, 301,* 114462. doi:10.1016/j. jviromet.2022.114462 PMID:35026305

Ge, Y., Tian, T., Huang, S., Wan, F., Li, J., Li, S., Wang, X., Yang, H., Hong, L., Wu, N., Yuan, E., Luo, Y., Cheng, L., Hu, C., Lei, Y., Shu, H., Feng, X., Jiang, Z., Wu, Y., ... Zeng, J. (2021). An integrative drug repositioning framework discovered a potential therapeutic agent targeting COVID-19. *Signal Transduction and Targeted Therapy, 6*(1), 165. doi:10.103841392-021-00568-6 PMID:33895786

Gifani, P., Shalbaf, A., & Vafaeezadeh, M. (2021). Automated detection of COVID-19 using ensemble of transfer learning with deep convolutional neural network based on CT scans. *International Journal of Computer Assisted Radiology and Surgery, 16*(1), 115–123. doi:10.100711548-020-02286-w PMID:33191476

Gil-Rodríguez, J., Pérez de Rojas, J., Aranda-Laserna, P., Benavente-Fernández, A., Martos-Ruiz, M., Peregrina-Rivas, J. A., & Guirao-Arrabal, E. (2022, March). Ultrasound findings of lung ultrasonography in COVID-19: A systematic review. *European Journal of Radiology*, *148*, 110156. doi:10.1016/j.ejrad.2022.110156 PMID:35078136

Global health, infectious disease, public health education. (2021, February 19). https://www.publichealth.columbia.edu/public-health-now/news/epidemic-endemic-pandemic-what-are-differences

Gudigar, A., Raghavendra, U., Nayak, S., Ooi, C. P., Chan, W. Y., Gangavarapu, M. R., Dharmik, C., Samanth, J., Kadri, N. A., Hasikin, K., Barua, P. D., Chakraborty, S., Ciaccio, E. J., & Acharya, U. R. (2021, December). Role of artificial intelligence in COVID-19 detection. *Sensors (Basel)*, *21*(23), 8045. doi:10.339021238045 PMID:34884045

Heidari, M., Mirniaharikandehei, S., Khuzani, A. Z., Danala, G., Qiu, Y., & Zheng, B. (2020). Improving the performance of CNN to predict the likelihood of COVID-19 using chest X-ray images with preprocessing algorithms. *International Journal of Medical Informatics*, *144*, 104284. doi:10.1016/j.ijmedinf.2020.104284 PMID:32992136

Heilweil, R. (n.d.). *How AI is battling the coronavirus Outbreak*. Available online: https://www.com/recode/2020/1/28/21110902/artificial-intelligence-ai-coronavirus-wuhan

Hemdan & Karar. (2020). *COVIDX-net: A framework of deep learning classifiers to diagnose COVID-19*. https://arxiv.org/abs/2003.11055

How are AI-based solutions being used to combat COVID-19? (n.d.). http://indiaai.gov.in/article/how-are-ai-based-solutions-bei ng-used-to-combat-covid-19

How India fights COVID with artificial intelligence. (2021). https://analyticsindiamag.com/how-india-fights-covid-with-artificial-intelligence/

Introduction to support vector machines (SVM). (n.d.). https://www.geeksforgeeks.org/introduction-to-support-vector-machines-svm/

K-nearest neighbor (KNN) algorithm for machine learning. (n.d.). https://www.javatpoint.com/k-nearest-neighbor-algorithm-for-machine-learning

Kajabad, E. N., & Ivanov, S. V. (2019). People detection and finding attractive areas by the use of movement detection analysis and deep learning approach. *Procedia Computer Science*, *156*, 327–337. doi:10.1016/j.procs.2019.08.209

Kaur, G., Tomar, P., & Singh, P. (2018). Design of cloud-based green IoT architecture for smart cities. In *Internet of things and big data analytics toward next-generation intelligence* (pp. 315–333). Springer., doi:10.1007/978-3-319-60435-0_13

Kernel, S. V. M. (n.d.). *Functions – 'Coz your SVM knowledge is incomplete without it*. https://techvidvan.com/tutorials/svm-kernel-functions/

Keshavarzi Arshadi, A., Webb, J., Salem, M., Cruz, E., Calad-Thomson, S., Ghadirian, N., Collins, J., Diez-Cecilia, E., Kelly, B., Goodarzi, H., & Yuan, J. S. (2020, August 18). Artificial intelligence for COVID-19 drug discovery and vaccine development. *Frontiers in Artificial Intelligence*, *3*, 65. doi:10.3389/frai.2020.00065 PMID:33733182

Khanna, V. V., Chadaga, K., Sampathila, N., Prabhu, S., Chadaga, R., & Umakanth, S. (2022). Diagnosing COVID-19 using artificial intelligence: A comprehensive review. *Network Modeling and Analysis in Health Informatics and Bioinformatics*, *11*(1), 25. doi:10.100713721-022-00367-1

Laguarta, J., Hueto, F., & Subirana, B. (2020). COVID-19 artificial intelligence diagnosis using only cough recordings. *IEEE Open Journal of Engineering in Medicine and Biology*, *1*, 275–281. doi:10.1109/OJEMB.2020.3026928 PMID:34812418

Lee, Y., Kim, Y. S., Lee, D. I., Jeong, S., Kang, G. H., Jang, Y. S., Kim, W., Choi, H. Y., Kim, J. G., & Choi, S. H. (2022). The application of a deep learning system developed to reduce the time for RT-PCR in COVID-19 detection. *Scientific Reports*, *12*(1), 1234. doi:10.103841598-022-05069-2 PMID:35075153

Lesson 1: Introduction to epidemiology. (n.d.). https://www.cdc.gov/csels/dsepd/ss1978/lesson1/section11.html

Li, M., Zhang, Z., Cao, W., Liu, Y., Du, B., Chen, C., Liu, Q., Uddin, M. N., Jiang, S., Chen, C., Zhang, Y., & Wang, X. (2020). Identifying novel factors associated with COVID-19 transmission and fatality using the machine learning approach. *The Science of the Total Environment*, *10*(764), 142810. doi:10.1016/j.scitotenv.142810 PMID:33097268

Li, X., Yu, J., Zhang, Z., Ren, J., Peluffo, A. E., Zhang, W., Zhao, Y., Wu, J., Yan, K., Cohen, D., & Wang, W. (2021). Network bioinformatics analysis provides insight into drug repurposing for COVID-19. *Medicine in Drug Discovery*, *10*, 100090. doi:10.1016/j.medidd.2021.100090 PMID:33817623

Liu, G., Carter, B., Bricken, T., Jain, S., Viard, M., Carrington, M., & Gifford, D. K. (2020). Computationally optimized SARS-CoV-2 MHC Class I and II Vaccine Formulations Predicted to Target Human Haplotype Distributions. *Cell Systems*, *11*(2), 131–144.e6. doi:10.1016/j.cels.2020.06.009 PMID:32721383

Liu, G., Carter, B., & Gifford, D. K. (2021). Predicted gaps for SARS-CoV-2 subunit vaccines and their augmentation by compact peptide sets. *Cell Systems*, *12*(1), 102–107.e4. doi:10.1016/j.cels.2020.11.010 PMID:33321075

Manfredi, M., Vezzani, R., Calderara, S., & Cucchiara, R. (2014). Detection of static groups and crowds gathered in open spaces by texture classification. *Pattern Recognition Letters*, *44*, 39–48. doi:10.1016/j.patrec.2013.11.001

Mankodiya, H., Palkhiwala, P., Gupta, R., Jadav, N. K., Tanwar, S., Neagu, B.-C., Grigoras, G., Alqahtani, F., & Shehata, A. M. (2022). A real-time CrowdsensingFramework for potential COVID-19 carrier detection using wearable sensors. *Mathematics*, *10*(16), 2927. doi:10.3390/math10162927

Martins, N. (n.d.). *How healthcare is using big data and AI to cure disease*. https://www.forbes.com/sites/nicolemartin1/2019/08/30/how-healthcare-is-using-big-data-and-ai-to-cure-disease/#7ebe957645cf

Matsuda, S., & Yoshimura, H. (2022). Personal identification with artificial intelligence under COVID-19 crisis: A scoping review. *Systematic Reviews*, *11*(1), 7. doi:10.118613643-021-01879-z PMID:34991695

Mukherjee, H., Ghosh, S., Dhar, A., Obaidullah, S. M., Santosh, K. C., & Roy, K. (2021). Deep neural network to detect COVID-19: One architecture for both CT Scans and Chest X-rays. *Applied Intelligence*, *51*(5), 2777–2789. doi:10.100710489-020-01943-6 PMID:34764562

Naïve Bayes classifier algorithm. (n.d.). https://www.javatpoint.com/machine-learning-naive-bayes-classifier

Narin, A., Kaya, C., & Pamuk, Z. (2021). Automatic detection of coronavirus disease (COVID-19) using X-ray images and deep convolutional neural networks. *Pattern Analysis & Applications*, *24*(3), 1207–1220. doi:10.100710044-021-00984-y PMID:33994847

Nayak, S. R., Nayak, D. R., Sinha, U., Arora, V., & Pachori, R. B. (2021, February). Application of deep learning techniques for detection of COVID-19 cases using chest X-ray images: A comprehensive study. *Biomedical Signal Processing and Control*, *64*, 102365. doi:10.1016/j.bspc.2020.102365 PMID:33230398

Nguyen, P. Q., Soenksen, L. R., Donghia, N. M., Angenent-Mari, N. M., de Puig, H., Huang, A., Lee, R., Slomovic, S., Galbersanini, T., Lansberry, G., Sallum, H. M., Zhao, E. M., Niemi, J. B., & Collins, J. J. (2021). Wearable materials with embedded synthetic biology sensors for biomolecule detection. *Nature Biotechnology*, *39*(11), 1366–1374. doi:10.103841587-021-00950-3 PMID:34183860

Ong, E., Wong, M. U., Huffman, A., & He, Y. (2020). COVID-19 coronavirus vaccine design using reverse vaccinology and machine learning. *Frontiers in Immunology*, *11*, 1581. doi:10.3389/fimmu.2020.01581 PMID:32719684

Özbilge, E., Sanlidag, T., Ozbilge, E., & Baddal, B. (2022). Artificial intelligence-assisted RT-PCR detection model for rapid and reliable diagnosis of COVID-19. *Applied Sciences (Basel, Switzerland)*, *12*(19), 9908. doi:10.3390/app12199908

Panwar, H., Gupta, P. K., Siddiqui, M. K., Morales-Menendez, R., & Singh, V. (2020). Application of deep learning for fast detection of COVID-19 in X-rays using nCOVnet. *Chaos, Solitons, and Fractals*, *138*, 109944. doi:10.1016/j.chaos.2020.109944 PMID:32536759

Pecoraro, V., Negro, A., Pirotti, T., & Trenti, T. (2022, February). Estimate false-negative RT-PCR rates for SARS-CoV-2. A systematic review and meta-analysis. *European Journal of Clinical Investigation*, *52*(2), e13706. doi:10.1111/eci.13706 PMID:34741305

Piret, J., & Boivin, G. (2020). Pandemics throughout history. *Frontiers in Microbiology*, *11*, 631736. doi:10.3389/fmicb.2020.631736 PMID:33584597

Principle component analysis. (n.d.). https://www.javatpoint.com/principal-component-analysis

Random forest algorithm. (n.d.). https://www.javatpoint.com/machine-learning-random-forest-algorithm

Rawat, K., Kumari, P., & Saha, L. (2021). COVID-19 vaccine: A recent update in pipeline vaccines, their design and development strategies. *European Journal of Pharmacology*, *892*, 173751. doi:10.1016/j.ejphar.2020.173751 PMID:33245898

Regression analysis in machine learning. (n.d.). https://www.javatpoint.com/regression-analysis-in-machine-learning

Statistical Language – Correlation and Causation at Australian Bureau of Statistics. (n.d.). https://www.abs.gov.au/

Stieg, C. (2020). *How this Canadian start-up spotted coronavirus before everyone else knew about it.* CNBC.

Sun, G., Matsui, T., Hakozaki, Y., & Abe, S. (2015). An infectious disease/fever screening radar system which stratifies higher-risk patients within ten seconds using a neural network and the fuzzy grouping method. *The Journal of Infection*, *70*(3), 230–236. doi:10.1016/j.jinf.2014.12.007 PMID:25541528

Support vector machine algorithm. (n.d.). https://www.javatpoint.com/machine-learning-support-vector-machine-algorithm

The, U. S. (2022, May 19). *Government and the World Health Organization*. https://www.kff.org/coronavirus-covid-19/fact-sheet/the-u-s-government-and-the-world-health-organization/

The Computer Algorithm That Was Among the First to Detect the Coronavirus Outbreak. (n.d.). http://www.cnbnews.com

Tomar, P., Kaur, G., & Singh, P. (2018). A prototype of IoT-based real time smart street parking system for smart cities. In *Internet of things and big data analytics toward next-generation intelligence* (pp. 243–263). Springer. doi:10.1007/978-3-319-60435-0_10

Tschoellitsch, T., Dünser, M., Böck, C., Schwarzbauer, K., & Meier, J. (2021, March). Machine learning prediction of SARS-CoV-2 polymerase chain reaction results with routine blood tests. *Laboratoriums Medizin 15, 52*(2), 146–149. doi:10.1093/labmed/lmaa111

Understanding random forest. (n.d.). https://www.analyticsvidhya.com/blog/2021/06/understanding-random-forest/

World Health Organization. (n.d.). *Coronavirus (COVID-19) dashboard*. https://covid19.who.int/table

Yadav, S., Gulia, P., Gill, N. S., & Chatterjee, J. M. (2022). A real-time crowd monitoring and management system for social distance classification and healthcare using deep learning. *Journal of Healthcare Engineering*. . doi:10.1155/2022/2130172

Zhong, F., Xing, J., Li, X., Liu, X., Fu, Z., Xiong, Z., Lu, D., Wu, X., Zhao, J., Tan, X., Li, F., Luo, X., Li, Z., Chen, K., Zheng, M., & Jiang, H. (2018). Artificial intelligence in drug design. *Science China. Life Sciences*, *61*(10), 1191–1204. doi:10.100711427-018-9342-2 PMID:30054833

Chapter 10
Cyberstalking:
Consequences and Coping Strategies to Improve Mental Health

Abhishek Bansal
Indira Gandhi National Tribal University, Amarkantak, India

Arvind Kumar Gautam
Indira Gandhi Naitonal Tribal University, Amarkantak, India

Sudesh Kumar
Indira Gandhi Naitonal Tribal University, Amarkantak, India

ABSTRACT

Cyberstalking is one of the most widespread threats on digital platforms. It has included many forms of direct threats via email, online distribution of intimate photographs, seeking information about victims, harassment, and catfishing. The consequences of cyberstalking may lead to psychological problems such as mental health, distress, victim experiencing feelings of isolation, guilt, adverse effects on life activity. These psychological problems may further lead to reports of serious health issues such as anger, fear, suicidal ideation, depression, and post-traumatic stress disorder (PTSD). However, there are many coping strategies such as avoidant coping, ignoring the perpetrator, confrontational coping, support seeking, and cognitive reframing. In spite of these methods, awareness of preventive measures of cyberstalking may further help to overcome mental stress. In this chapter, the authors have pointed out the various psychological issues due to cyberstalking and further discuss their solutions through preventing or automatic detection methods inspired by machine learning approaches.

DOI: 10.4018/978-1-6684-6646-9.ch010

INTRODUCTION

Virtual stalking is a new form of cybercrime due to the advancement of the virtual platform for social activities. As per the Statista (2021a) report published on August 17, 2021, India had more than 749 million internet users across the country in 2020. Most of the Internet users in India access the internet to visit social media sites like YouTube, Facebook, Twitter, Instagram, Linkedin, Telegram, and many more. These sites have different types of content which are created by the users. These contents may include personal details, pictures, family videos, family relationships, private chats, and financial information. Cybercriminals have exploited this information to perform cybercriminal activities like stalking, bullying, and cyber fraud.

Cyberstalking is a social, psychological, and criminal issue that is liable for a fierce and criminal society, particularly among students and women of different organisations. Cyberstalking and cyberbullying are much similar content-wise and intent-wise, which utilise internet technology and similar approaches to follow or target someone in the web-based world. There is no universally accepted definition of cyberstalking. The word stalking means 'pursue stealthily,' which refers that "harass obviously." It is the use of the internet or other electronic means to stalk or harass a person. The utilisation of technology allows stalkers to harass their targets from any part of the world. Cyberstalking is nothing but online harassment, threatening the victim for sexual purposes or misusing them. Some scholars said that "Cyberstalking and Cyberbullying are often used interchangeably and involve using the internet to stalk or target someone in the online world," while some scholars explore that "Cyberstalking is a form of cyberbullying with many similarities. "Cyberstalking is the use of the internet or other electronic means to stalk or harass any individual, group, or organisation. Cyberstalking may also include monitoring, identity theft, threats, vandalism, doxing, blackmail, solicitation for sex, or gathering information that may be used to threaten or harass. Many scholars have defined cyberstalking as one of the most dangerous forms of cyber harassment. Cyberstalkers use online web media and other electronic devices with pre-plans and agendas to follow, undermine, and harass others, as shown in Figure 1.

Cyberstalking is a growing and tangled cybercrime that influences and intentions of individuals and groups (Baer M., 2020). Cyberstalking is intensely planned, repeated, and different advanced attacks and may occur on repeated occurrences (Truman J. L., 2010). There are various examples of cyberstalking, such as creating and sharing sexual images of the victim among their family and friends, hacking the victim's social media and email accounts, and transferring the victim's private data on social media (N. M. Zainudin et al., 2016). Savaging and flaring to somebody in the web-based network, making counterfeit profiles, tracking internet activities through tracking devices, making fake messages intended to shame victim, offering

Figure 1. Cyberstalker and victim

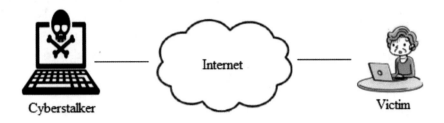

an unwanted gift, mobbing utilising rehashed messages, stigmatising somebody, sharing and trip the private information of somebody in a web-based application, annoying consistently, and hacking the casualty records and gadgets are some latest examples of cyberstalking.

Based on the technology involved, cyberstalking may be categorised into the following types (Ogilvie E., 2000).

- **Email stalking:** Email stalking occurs in the email network by sending content containing phishing, viruses, threatening, fraudulent, and harassing content, email bombing, as well as sharing the private information of victims.
- **Internet stalking:** Internet stalking occurs on online media applications through fake or real accounts to harass and undermine the victim on social media platforms.
- **Computer stalking:** Computer stalking utilises several types of attacks on the computerless of the victim to theft and destroys data.
- **Phone stalking:** When stalkers harass the victim by utilising a phone through phone calls, or messages in a repeated manner, it is called phone stalking.
- **Automated stalking:** Automatic cyberstalking is a cutting-edge approach used by cyberstalkers to target casualties using automatic computer programs and mobile apps operated through suspicious servers.

Cyberstalking act is performed by the attacker known as a stalker. Muller et al. (1999) studied 145 stalkers who received treatment in a forensic psychiatry centre. Based on his study, Muller has categorised different kinds of a stalker as follows.

- **Rejected Stalker:** A person who feels insulted by friends and organisations. They act stalking to reconcile damaged self-respect and feel happy from an act of cyberstalking.

- **Intimacy Stalker:** This stalker performs cyberstalking to gain information or attract the opposite sex for the purpose of love and intimacy. This type of stalker has an introverted personality.
- **Incompetent Stalker:** This stalker also acts cyberstalking to establish an affair relationship. They want to try to find a date or a sexual encounter.
- **Resentful Stalker:** This type of stalker wants to take revenge. They feel satisfied by harm to their target.
- **Predatory Stalker:** The purpose of a predatory stalker is to search such victims who are ready for sex. The purpose of this type of stalking is to fulfil the need for sex. They try to find the personal detail of the victim, and based on that detail, they blackmail and force them to make a relationship with him.
- **Collective Stalker:** These stalkers are in groups and act collectively. The main target of this group is business organisations and government organisations.

In spite of the above stalker, stalkers may also have categories for stealing banking information for financial fraud, stealing passwords to unlock social media accounts, and harming the image of a famous person. Several pieces of research show that cyberstalkers also suffer from mental problems (Khader, M. et al., 2020). Cyberstalkers may be categorised into different types based on their mental conditions (Kamphuis, J. H. et al., 2000). The common obsession stalker refuses to believe that their relationship is over. The delusional stalker may have a mental illness like schizophrenia and assume that the victim loves them even though they have never met. They are challenging to shake off. The vengeful stalker is angry at their victim for some minor personal reason, either real or imagined. Cyberstalking is one kind of interpersonal violence and a major factor affecting victims' mental health. Cyberstalking is often underestimated by society, researchers, and public authorities. The consequences of cyberstalking may lead to psychological problems such as mental health, distress, victim experiencing feelings of isolation, guilt, and adverse effects on life activities such as social relationships and occupational activity, and irritability (Begotti, T et al., 2020 & Acquadro Maran et al., 2019).

Recently, many cyberstalking and other cyber harassment cases have been reported in India. As per NCRB report 2020, Vol.2, chapter 9A (https://www.thehinducentre. com, 2020), the number of cybercrime cases, as shown in Table 1, was registered in various states of India under Information Technology Act from 2018 to 2020.

As per the statistics of cybercrime cases, UP, Karnataka, Maharashtra, Telangana & Assam are the most affected states by cybercrime. The NCRB report may further categorise different kinds of cybercrime registered under the IT Act 2008 (https:// police.py.gov.in). These crimes are shown in Table 2.

As per the report, the cause of cybercrime are personal revenge, anger, fraud, extortion, causing disrepute, prank, sexual exploitation, political motives, terrorist

Table 1. Cyber Crimes (State / UT- wise during 2018 to 2020)

State/States/UTs	Cases Registered		
	2018	2019	2020
Uttar Pradesh	6280	11416	11097
Karnataka	5839	12020	10741
Maharashtra	3511	4967	5496
Telangana	1205	2691	5024
Assam	2022	2231	3530
Odisha	843	1485	1931
Andhra Pradesh	1207	1886	1899
Bihar	374	1050	1512
Rajasthan	1104	1762	1354
Gujarat	702	784	1283
Jharkhand	930	1095	1204
Tamil Nadu	295	385	782
West Bengal	335	524	712
Madhya Pradesh	740	602	699
Haryana	418	564	656
Kerala	340	307	426
Punjab	239	243	378
Chhattisgarh	139	175	297
Delhi	189	115	168
Uttarakhand	171	100	143
Meghalaya	74	89	142
Jammu & Kashmir	73	73	120
Himachal Pradesh	69	76	98
Manipur	29	4	79
Goa	29	15	40
Tripura	20	20	34
Arunachal Pradesh	7	8	30
Chandigarh	30	23	17
Mizoram	6	8	13
Puducherry	14	4	10
Nagaland	2	2	8
A&N Islands	7	2	5
Lakshadweep	4	4	3
Daman & Diu	0	3	3
Ladakh	0	0	1
Sikkim	1	2	0

Table 2. Cyber Crimes under various sections of IT Act 2008 (registered in States/UTs)

Cyber Crimes Registered in India	IT Act 2008
Tampering Computer Source documents	Section 65
Ransomware	Section 66
Dishonestly receiving stolen computer resources or communication device	Section 66 B
Identity Theft	Section 66 C
Cheating by personation by using computer resource	Section 66 D
Violation of Privacy	Section 66 E
Cyber Terrorism	Section 66 F
Publication/ transmission of obscene / sexually explicit act in electronic form	Section 67 A
Publishing or transmitting of material depicting children in the Sexually explicit act in electronic form	Section 67 B
Preservation and retention of information by Intermediaries	Section 67 C
Interception or monitoring or decryption of Information	Section 69
Unauthorised access/attempt to access protected computer system	Section 70
Abetment of Suicide (Online)	Section 305/306 IPC
Cyber Stalking/ Bullying of Women/ Children	Section 354 D IPC
Data theft	Section 379 to 381
Fraud (ATM, Online banking, OTP and others)	Section 420 r/w Section 465, 468-471 IPC
Forgery	Sections 465,468 & 471
Fake Profile	r/w IPC/SLL
Cyber Blackmailing/ Threatening	Section 506,503,384 IPC
Fake News on Social Media	Section 505
Insult the modesty of any Woman	Section 509

activities like recruitment and funding, inciting hatred against the country, disrupting public service, sales purchase the illegal drug, spreading piracy, stealing information, and abetment of suicide. Cybercriminals mainly target women on social media platforms. As per the NCRB 2020 report, there were several cases registered against women in 2020. The main causes of these cases are cyber blackmailing, cyber pornography/ publishing obscene sexual materials, cyberstalking and cyberbullying, defamation, and fake profiling. In the case of cyberstalking and cyberbullying against women, the most affected states are shown in Figure 2.

Figure 2. States which reported the highest number of cases of cyberstalking and cyberbullying against women in 2020

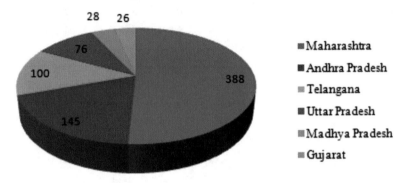

RECENT REPORTED CYBERSTALKING CASES IN INDIA

In India, the first case of CyberStalking (Prakash R., 2019) was reported in 2000, wherein the crime branch arrested Manish Kathuria, who was stalking a woman by illegally chatting on the chat website mIRC using her name. He distributed her mobile number and invited her to chat on her phone; as a result, women received so many anonymous calls from different places. Women got disturbed mentally and filed a complaint to Delhi Police. The police department registered this case under section 509 of the IPC for outraging the modesty of a woman.

On July 4, 2015, Hindustan Times published a report (https://www.hindustantimes. com, 2015), "35-year-old first convict in a cyberstalking case in Maharashtra". As per that report, a 35-year-old, Yogesh Prabhu convicted under section 509 and section E of the IT Act 2008. Yogesh has been sentenced to three months of simple imprisonment and fined 10000 for the offence of sending obscene pictures and videos via email to a woman who he met on social media. On September 7, 2020, The Indian Express reported a cyberstalking case (https://indianexpress.com/article/cities/delhi/ghaziabad-man -held-for-stalking-harassing-women-6585841/) of a Ghaziabad man who was found to harass more than 500 women using software to make calls that would mask his mobile number. As per police, he allegedly dialled different combinations of mobile numbers, and if the woman picked up, he would save the number and send lewd messages on WhatsApp chats. A lawyer filed his complaint, and the cyber cell team traced his IP address and arrested him. On April 6, 2021, the Times of India published a report (https://timesofindia.indiatimes.com/life-style/spotlight/bew are-cyberstalking-is-on-the-rise-during-the-pandemic/article show/81924158.cms) on "Beware! Cyberstalking is on the rise during the pandemic". In this report, a new cyberstalking case has been described. In this case, a Pune-based Archeology student noticed that a random account liked almost 200 pictures of hers on Instagram. She ignored it as harmless until the stalker started posting lewd messages on her account. Stalker then started sending her direct message asking "if she would like to go on a date with him". Again, she ignored them, but the stalker started abusing language and threatening to make her his wife forcefully. The student got mentally disturbed and registered an online complaint with the cyber police. On April 28, 2021, The Times of India reported a new cyberstalking incident (https://timesofindia.indiatimes.com/city/hyderabad/two-arres ted-for-cyber-stalking/articleshow/82280780.cms) from Hyderabad. In this case, Rachakonda cyber crime police arrested two people in a separate incident for allegedly stalking the victim on a social media platform and sending an obscene message. In the first case, a 25-year-old person created a fake Facebook profile using a virtual phone number and sent sexual content to his colleague to disturb her marital relationship. In another case, a private employee was convicted of sending sexually explicit content to a minor girl he met on a fake profile on Instagram.

On January 3, 2022, Zee News published a report on the Bulli Bai controversy (https://zeenews.india.com/india/bulli-bai-controversy-all-yo u-need-to-know-about-the-app-targeting-muslim-women-on-socia l-media-2424831.html). Bulli Bai and Sulli Deals sites are the latest examples of cyber harassment against women. Bulli Bai is the clone website of Sulli deals which was uploaded on GitHub. In this case, the website owner allegedly uploaded photos of women for auction without their consent. The site owner would use the photos from social media sites and promote them on Twitter to convince people to participate in the auction. These sites have been created on the GitHub platform. The Information & Technology minister has filed a complaint against the site owner under section 509 in the cyber police station of Delhi police.

The above cyberstalking cases show that cyberstalking, cyberbullying, and cyber blackmailing are serious issues that cause mental stress to the victim and their families.

CONSEQUENCES OF CYBERSTALKING

Cyberstalking is not only a crime, but it leads to mental stress for the victims. It has major psychosocial impacts such as fear, confusion, anger, anxiety, insomnia, and post-traumatic stress disorder (PTSD). PTSD disorder includes re-experience symptoms like upsetting memories, flashbacks, nightmares, emotional and physical reactions, change in thinking and mood, negative thoughts, blaming yourself, feeling detached, feeling irritable, angry outbursts, and sleeping problems. As per Statistica (2021b), 518 million people in India have social media profiles in which people share personal information with each other. They also used chat boxes to share personal feelings. Sometimes this information is leaked or stalked by family members like spouses, co-workers, and close friends. Therefore, the victims felt various mental and emotional health issues like shame, guilt, anger, self-blame, and fear. In some cases, married couples destroy their married life due to frequently stalking their spouse's social media accounts. It leads to mental stress due to cyberstalking.

Many articles have been published on the impact of mental health due to cyberstalking, cyber harassment, and cyberbullying in the literature. Most of the articles are based on either survey of college students or review papers published in previous years. Some articles have been discussed in this chapter to understand the consequences of cyberstalking. Stevens F. et al. (2021) published a review paper in which more than 1077 available articles based on the impact of cyber abuse on mental health are analysed. He found that email, Facebook, text messages, classroom, blogs, GPS applications such as "Find my friends," and social media sites like Whatsapp, WebChat, BeeTalk, Viber, Telegram, tumbler, and Youtube are the main source in which cyber hackers are active. He also found that most cyberstalking victims have experienced emotional and mental consequences like depression, fear, anxiety, stress/PTSD, anger, self-harm, embarrassment, isolation, panic, sadness, paranoia, and fear. The criteria for measuring emotional and mental disorders are based on a survey of the participants, participant's experience, general health questionnaires, the WHO-5 well-being index, the symptom checklist-90-R, the back depression inventory II, and the Hopkins symptoms checklist. Villora B. et al. (2020) presented a study on the association between bullying and well-being dimensions (emotional, social, and psychological) among university students who are victims of cyberdating abuse and bullying. In this study, approximately 1657 university students have participated, and based on their experiences, the researcher has analysed the association through various statistical methods like multiple regression and ANCOVA analysis. In his study, the researcher found that bullying victimisation could significantly affect university students, especially in well-being dimensions such as emotional, social, and psychological.

Melander LA et al. (2020) and Kawan et al. (2020) and investigated the relationship between cyberbullying and mental outcomes among young people. The methodology of this study is based on preferred reporting items for systematic reviews and meta-analysis (PRISRM) guidance. The outcomes of this study confirm the strong negative relationship between cyberbullying and mental and psychosocial health. Bigotti et al. (2019) have performed a study to compare victims of one type of cyberstalking with victims who have suffered more than one type of cyberstalking. In this study, victims have responded to their mental experience in terms of physical, emotional, depression, and anxiety symptoms, as shown in Figure 3.

In this study, researchers found that more than half of the participants had experienced at least one cyberstalking incident. 14.6 percent of victims have suffered from headaches and tiredness, and 12.2 percent have experienced sleep disorder, nausea, panic attack, and weakness in the case of physical symptoms. Similarly, 37.3 percent of victims who experienced more than one cyberstalking have suffered from a sleep disorder, while 28.8% have suffered from tiredness. In the case of emotional symptoms, 56.1% of the victims have suffered from anger, while 48.8 percent suffered from irritation. Moreover, 58.1% have suffered from depression, and 42.8 percent have experienced anxiety.

The above literature shows the adverse effect on the mental condition of cyber victims. Victims are suffering or stressed by the stalker and feel different kinds of symptoms. They are as follows-

- Mental health symptoms include self-doubt, wondering, over-reacting, confusion and denial, frustration, embarrassment, self-blame, sleep disorder, panic attacks, insecurity, suicidal thoughts, and self-medication.
- Effect on school or work as leaving a job, sick leave, changing jobs, dropping school, and deteriorating work/school performance.
- Effect on social life, such as problems in emotional and physical intimacy, isolation, changing contact numbers or moving to a new place, and insecurity.

Figure 3. Cyberstalking consequences

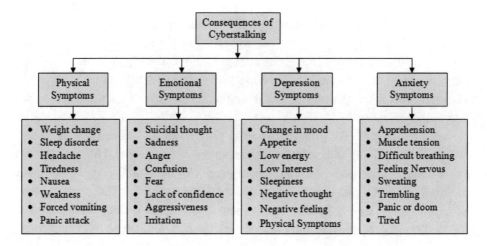

- Effect on finance as loss of wages cost spent in legal fees, expenses, cost spent on medical treatment and expanses to seeking psychological counselling.

COPING STRATEGY TO IMPROVE MENTAL HEALTH

Online namelessness makes it try to follow cyberstalking back to a specific individual. However, there is still some strategy to combat cyberstalking. In the literature, several techniques are suggested by researchers to cope with cyberstalking. This strategy is based on a psychological or emotional strategy as well as a problem-solving coping strategy. The most common techniques to reduce stress in psychology are avoidant coping, ignoring the perpetrator, confrontational coping, support seeking, and cognitive reframing.

- **Avoidant Coping:** Avoidant coping is the strategy in which the victim may avoid online activities in which they have had a bad experience in the past. If the victim suffers from a specific relative or friend on social media, they must unfriend that person.
- **Ignoring the Perpetrator:** Sometimes ignoring is the best strategy to cope with various frauds. A victim is involved in a relationship with a social media friend without knowing his history. Therefore, this leads to increased mental stress. So the best strategy is to ignore activities sent by an unknown person.
- **Confrontational Coping:** Confrontational coping involves an aggressive reaction of altering the situation or forgiveness that is important to interpersonal relationships. Extensive use of social media sites may lead to stress among friends or relatives due to stalking. Therefore, the confrontational coping strategy may help to reduce stress.
- **Support Seeking:** Social support is much helpful in managing stress from any mental issues. Therefore, victims can overcome their stress with discussion or support from their parents, friends, and psychological experts.
- **Cognitive Reframing:** Positive environment and positive people are important to overcome mental stress for cyber victims. Therefore, cognitive reframing can play an important role in making the environment positive. In this approach, experts tried to reframe the negative emotion to position emotion. Eg. The negative thought, as I am stuck at home, can be reframed as I am safe at home. Similarly, the negative phrase "My friend and I can not see each other" can turn into positive phrases such as "My friend and I are protecting each other."

The psychological coping strategy helps to reduce mental stress up to some extent. In addition to these methods, experts have proposed prevention and detection coping approaches to surf the internet safely. They are as follows.

Cyberstalking Prevention Approaches

Cyberstalking prevention approaches are aware that users avoid cyberstalking cases. The primary step to addressing cyberstalking is to stop cooperation with the cyberstalker. While cyberstalkers often try to track down alternate ways of contacting the victims. Some barriers must be set up from the user end to stop cyberstalking. Another way to avoid cyberstalking is to increase the security of personal accounts in social media and other web-based applications. It's memorable that individuals who participate in cyberstalking are now crossing various individual limits to connect with the user. Thus, users should do all that to build online security. Substantial barriers and robust protection of personal accounts are not always enough to combat cyberstalkers. If victims feel that cyberstalkers are targeting them, then decisive action against cyberstalkers is required to cope with the cyberstalking. Experts and researchers suggest following some basic prevention guidelines to avoid and adequately handle cyberstalking.

- **Strictly warn cyberstalkers to stop cyberstalking:** In the initial stage of cyberstalking, users should strictly warn cyberstalkers to stop cyberstalking. Nothing more replies or explanations are required from the user's end.
- **Block the cyberstalker:** After a strict warning, users should immediately block that suspicious person from all social media accounts, mobile phones, and other internet applications.
- **Do not reply to cyberstalkers:** Suppose the cyberstalkers are continuing to target the victim and try to connect and ask or demand some things. In that case, users should ignore and do not respond to anything against the post, messages, or emails of cyberstalkers.
- **Change personal account and lock the profile:** Suppose users' personal accounts or email IDs are well known to cyberstalkers. In that case, users should change email ids, change personal accounts, change display names and profile pictures and finally, lock the social media account for other than friends.
- **Make a strong password and change it regularly:** Cyberstalkers often try to hack the personal accounts of users. To avoid this situation, users should change their passwords regularly and make them more potent.

- **Avoid the overuse of online accounts:** As far as possible, avoid the overuse of social media accounts and do not share private pictures. If still facing the cyberstalking issue, take a long break from social media accounts.
- **Use proper antivirus and uninstall any suspicious or unknown apps:** Cyberstalkers often use mobile apps and other web-based applications to steal confidential information from user's devices. Users should install proper antivirus and uninstall any suspicious and unknown apps from the device.
- **Make documentation of cyberstalking as evidence:** If the user feels that someone has cyberstalked them, they should immediately verify cyberstalking activities as evidence.
- **Report cyberstalking case to the police station:** After having sufficient evidence or without any evidence, the victim should immediately report to the police station regarding cyberstalking. In case of not proper reporting by the victim, cyberstalkers often become more dangerous and perform cyberstalking continually.

Automatic Cyberstalking Detection Approaches

Prevention approaches are suitable for general awareness about cyberstalking, and their proper use may avoid the circumstances of cyberstalking to certain limits. Efficient automated cyberstalking detection and controlling strategies should be used on the user and application end to cope with the cyberstalking properly. Researchers have suggested several automatic detections and controlling techniques to combat cyberstalking on different virtual world platforms. Researchers have utilised machine learning, data mining, deep learning, fuzzy logic, and neural network techniques either as a single or hybrid approach to developing automatic detection and control models against cyberstalking. Several researchers have also implemented the detection model in different languages to cope with cyberstalking and other cyberharassment. Text-based, image-based, audio-based, and video-based detection techniques have been introduced by several researchers on various platforms of the virtual world.

Cyberstalking Detection Techniques

Cyberstalkers utilise their own internet-based innovative methodology with certain plans, groups, and agendas to target the victims and accomplish their objectives. Researchers are fostering the cyberstalking identification model involving several detection techniques for fighting stalkers. In the literature, various primary and supporting techniques have been utilised either as single or hybrid approaches (Figure 4) for cyberstalking and related cybercrime detection (W. A. Al-Khater et al., 2020).

Figure 4. Several techniques for cyberstalking and other cyberharassment detection

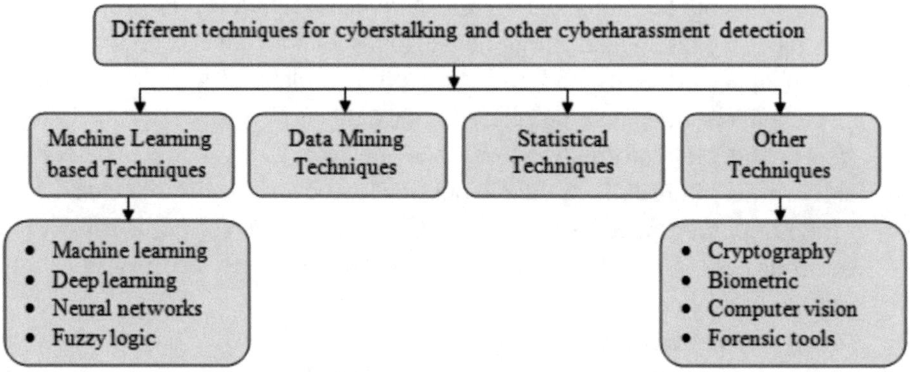

Cyberstalking Detection Utilising Machine Learning (ML)

Researchers broadly utilise machine Learning-based techniques for cyberstalking detection and control on different platforms of social media and other virtual world applications. Various techniques of machine learning are used as a single approach and a hybrid approach. Neural networks, deep learning, and fuzzy logic approaches, a subset of machine learning, are widely utilised to enhance the performance of detection models on large and complex datasets (Tobla et al., 2021, Sadiq S., 2021, & Ayo F., 2021). Neural network-based techniques can prepare and learn without and are suitable for performing computations faster because they work like the human mind. Deep learning is a three-layer-based subset of machine learning. Deep learning can update and refine for precision on large and complex datasets. Fuzzy logic is a figuring method that contains conventional and fuzzy sets, and it works by relying upon the degree of truth as opposed to boolean logic (Bini et al., 2018).

Cyberstalking Detection Utilising Data Mining

Data mining is a more manual cycle that relies upon human intervention and procedure. Initially, advances in the approach to data mining, rules, or models are obscure, and it uses the current dataset as a data warehouse to find plans (Singhal et al., 2013).

Cyberstalking Detection Utilising Statistical Method

The researchers propose some statistically based techniques for cyberstalking and other kinds of cyberharassment identification (Tolba et al., 2021). For example, the CPRA-EWMA, CPRA-Shewhart, Hidden Markov Model, Bayesian learning network approach, and anomaly detection calculation are useful for cyberstalking detection model.

Cyberstalking Detection Utilising Other Techniques

Some different strategies like Cryptography, biometrics, Computer Vision, and Forensics Tools are likewise involved by researchers for cyberstalking and other cyberharassment identification and proof collections. Cyberstalking detection utilising the cryptography approach focuses on verifying and checking the cyberstalker's identity and the main source of cyberstalking information. A biometric framework is mainly a supportive tool in face recognition, picture distinguishing proof, and stalker verification. Computer vision strategies examine the images and decide if URLs are certifiable or counterfeit. Crime scene investigation devices manage the assortment of evidence from computerised media, and it is helpful to follow the activities of cyberstalkers and address security issues (Derhab A., 2014 & Peters, J. F., 2017).

Several cyberstalking detection models using several cyberstalking detection techniques are suggested and implemented by the researchers in the literature. Text-based cyberstalking and cyberbullying detection techniques proposed and tested by Dinakar K., 2011 Soundar K., 2016; Raisi E., 2016; Ptaszynski M., 2016; Nahar V., 2014; H. Li, 2016; Galan-Garcia P., 2016, Dadvar M., 2012.

These researchers utilised various machine learning techniques to implement the detection model on several datasets (Twitter, Youtube, Facebook, Instagram, etc.) and achieved better accuracy. Further developed identification strategies proposed by Ghasem Z. et al. (2015) involve machine learning techniques for controlling cyberbullying and cyberstalking. This methodology is predominantly centred around automatic detection and evidence documentation of email-based cyberstalking. The authors used machine learning, data mining, factual analysis, and email crime scene investigation to recognise and ease email-based cyberstalking. The authors tested the experimental work, including support vector machine and neural network strategies, in 5172 spam and non-spam email datasets. Frommholz I. et al. (2016) proposed a more improved text-based detection and cyberstalking control method using machine learning techniques. The author's proposed approaches revolved around maker ID, message order, personalisation, and computerised message legal sciences.

In 2021, Asante et al. (2021) implemented an enhanced technical solution for coping with content-based cyberstalking. The authors claimed that the proposed framework could automatically detect cyberstalking and provide the necessary support for law enforcement. The author's framework can identify the message, filter and detect the content, and collect the required evidence against cyberstalkers. Machine learning, data mining, and forensics tools were utilised to implement the proposed detection model. Another automatic detection model was proposed by kumar A. et al. (2021) to cope with cyberstalkers on social media. The authors developed a hybrid model using deep learning techniques and found better results. Another deep learning-based model was proposed by Alotaibi et al. (2021) to identify and detect harmful, abusive, aggressive, and offensive content on social media. Gautam et al. (2023) also proposed a real-time automatic cyberstalking detection model on Twitter, utilising a hybrid approach and found better results. Continually, authors Jadhav et al. (2021) developed a cyber safety model against abusive content on social media. The author's model can automatically detect cyberbullying and cyberstalking-related posts. Another real-time detection model suggested by authors Rizwan et al. (2021) for combating the different types of cyberharassment on social media. Machine learning techniques were utilised to implement the proposed model. In 2022, Gautam et al. (2022) reviewed several cyberstalking detection techniques. They found that machine learning and natural language processing play an important role in cyberstalking detection on different platforms of the internet world. Gautam et al. (2022) proposed and tested a cyberstalking detection model using machine learning techniques. The authors measured the performance of several machine learning classifiers on different sizes of datasets and found better results. Gautam et al. (2022) proposed another model for cyberstalking detection using machine learning classifiers with several features extraction techniques (Bag of Word, TF-IDF, Word2Vec, GloVe, FastText, ELMo, and BERT). In the experimental results, the authors found that the feature extraction technique is a significant factor in enhancing the performance of cyberstalking detection. The author's experimental results suggested that traditional feature extraction techniques outperformed advanced word embedding-based and language model-based feature extraction techniques with machine learning classifiers. As a real-time automated cyberstalking detection over email platform, Gautam et al. (2023) proposed an improved model for automatic detection of cyberstalking email through textual content and a basic intent-wise approach of cyberstalkers. The authors utilised the multi-model soft voting technique of machine learning to design and develop their proposed model EBCD (Email Based Cyberstalking Detection). EBCD model can automatically classify the emails from the user's mailbox into cyberstalking, suspicious, and normal emails and finally automatically move the classified emails to a particular folder.

Methodology Used in Automatic Cyberstalking Detection

The automatic cyberstalking detection model utilises several phases to detect cyberstalking. Data collection and preparing the datasets, pre-processing, feature extraction, cyberstalking detection, evidence collection, and performance measurement are essential phases used in the cyberstalking detection model. A training and testing dataset is initially cleaned and prepared through natural language processing pre-processing techniques. Several steps of the pre-processing methods, namely removal of stop words, noise removal, normalisation, tokenisation, Stemming, and Lemmatization, are crucial to enhance cyberstalking detection performance.

Another essential phase in cyberstalking detection is feature extraction. Feature extraction methods convert the text data of the dataset into feature vectors in a numerical form so that machine learning algorithms can be trained and tested on the dataset. In Figure 5, a machine learning-based methodology for cyberstalking identification is described.

Data Collection and Preparing the Datasets

Data collection and preparing the datasets are required in any methodology of cyberstalking detection. Some related datasets are initially ready to train the machine learning classifiers in this phase. As per the nature of machine learning algorithms, proper training of classifiers through sufficient and accurate training datasets is required before applying machine learning classifiers to actual data for cyberstalking detection. The performance of the cyberstalking detection model is much dependent on the different aspects of datasets. The source of the dataset (such as Twitter, Facebook, YouTube, Instagram, Email, etc.), size and distribution of the dataset (small, medium, and large), and accuracy of the labelled dataset are

Figure 5. Methodology for automatic cyberstalking detection using a machine learning approach

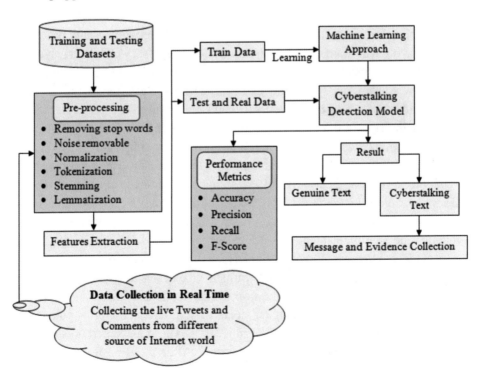

some essential factors that should be appropriately analysed before training to any classifiers with the selected datasets. After making the training and testing datasets, efficient algorithms are required to fetch the actual data from different sources of the internet world to apply the trained machine learning classifiers for cyberstalking identification and evidence collection. The data fetching algorithms are designed according to cyberstalking platforms, although different cyberstalking platforms have some limitations also in fetching the data in real-time. Twitter, Facebook, Instagram, and other social media applications provide an API-based facility to collect data in just real-time while posting tweets and comments by cyberstalkers. In the case of email-based cyberstalking and phone-based cyberstalking (WhatsApp and other similar cyberstalking apps), collecting the data in real-time is not possible through API on the researcher's end due to the privacy policy of service providers. This limitation of service providers raises cyberstalking cases quickly and increases the confidence of cyberstalkers to target the victims. Making the datasets containing fake accounts, profiles of identified cyberstalkers, and other cybercriminals active on social media and other internet applications is another challenging task in collecting and preparing the datasets. After rectifying all discussed issues and parameters, prepared datasets and actual data collected through different sources of internet applications are sent to pre-processing phase for cleaning the data.

Pre-Processing

Datasets gathered from different sources of social networks, and other web applications often contain different pointless and unnecessary characters, symbols, or text. Before assessing the machine learning algorithms, cleaned and arranged information are obligatory for the machine learning classifier in the detection stage. Data from the datasets are separated and standardised to a particular format. Pre-processing steps are required because they often enhance the performance of the cyberstalking detection model. In the pre-processing stage, generally, different tasks are performed utilising Natural Language Processing (NLP) according to the language of the text. Some useful pre-processing tasks include stop words expulsion tasks, noise removal, standardisation, tokenisation, stemming, and lemmatisation. In the datasets, common words that don't give meaning and don't decide syntactic, semantic, and sentiment meanings are called stop words (Vijayarani, S., 2015). Any articles, pronouns, prepositions, and so on in the datasets are examples of stop words. Algorithms to remove the stop words from datasets are designed according to the language used in the text. Like stop words, the dataset also contains various unnecessary special characters, digits, pieces of text, repeated words, punctuation marks, and white spaces in the form of noise data. These unwanted noise data are also required to be removed from the datasets. After these basic steps, another required pre-processing task is used to split the sentences into words. The process of splitting the sentences into words and stored into a separate list is called tokenisation. Datasets often contain both forms of data as lowercase and uppercase letters and need to be normalised into lowercase or uppercase letters for uniformity. Converting the digits into equivalent letters and converting all text into lower case letters or upper case letters is called normalisation. The normalisation process is highly needed because words with the same meaning as 'book' and 'BOOK' will explain non-similar words in the dataset and raises an extra burden for the feature extraction process. Generally, users prefer to convert all text to lowercase letters during normalisation. Datasets also often contain many repeated words of similar meanings, which are required to remove utilising the stemming and lemmatisation process. These processes support reducing the unnecessary computation of words. A method of changing all related words (related with different tense forms) to their root word is called stemming (Kadhim et al., 2018). Stemming offers vital help to dispense with undesirable computation of words from the dataset. For example, 'ride', 'rode', and 'ridden' will be changed over into 'ride' utilising streaming strategies. Lemmatisation is an alternative method of stemming which merges several related words into a single word and removes other related words using the synonyms of the words existing in the language. In this process, synonyms of each related word with similar meanings are determined, and one word is selected for the list while other words of similar purposes are removed from the list. Lemmatisation utilises the part of speech and lexicon-based dictionaries in natural language processing. Stemming is a simpler process than lemmatisation, although lemmatisation may be a better choice in the case of morphological analysis of words. Lemmatization is a more accurate but slower and more intensive process than steaming. Stemming might be more valuable in inquiries for data sets, while lemmatisation might work much better in the case of text sentiment analysis. All processing tasks (Removing Stop words, Noise Removal, Tokenisation, Normalisation, Stemming, and Lemmatization) are generally unnecessary in all cases. Pre-processing tasks are, moreover, liable for expanding or diminishing the performance of machine learning classifiers. Determination of pre-processing process according to datasets, languages, and features extraction models. After performing the pre-processing task, cleaned and formatted information is sent for feature extraction.

Features Extraction

In this stage of cyberstalking detection model, texts of datasets are converted into a numerical form using the feature extraction methods because machine learning classifiers can not understand the data as text form directly. The feature extraction method is required in the machine learning-based cyberstalking detection model. It utilised a feature dictionary and prepared a feature vector to convert the textual data into numerical data. Feature extraction techniques are a crucial factor in improving the performance of machine learning classifiers in cyberstalking detection. Feature extraction finds the weights of the words in the text and afterwards makes a feature vector as per the gathering of predefined keywords and dictionaries. Feature extraction methods utilise filtration, fusion, mapping, and clustering techniques to determine the feature vector. The filtration technique depends on word recurrence, data gain, and shared data. Fusion strategies utilise the joining of explicit classifiers for feature extraction. Clustering methods consider the basic similarity of text to cluster text features. Mapping strategies are broadly utilised for feature extraction, which utilises the LSI (dormant semantic file) and PCA (Principal Component Analysis) procedures. In the literature, researchers are using several basic and modern feature extraction to enhance the performance of the cyberstalking detection model. Bag of Words, TF-IDF, Word2Vec, GloVe, FastText, ELMo, BERT, ALBERT, ELECTRA, GPT-2, XLNET, Roberta, SBERT, Doc2VEC, InferSent, and Universal Sentence Encoder are a few well-known classical, word embedding based and language model-based feature extraction models that are frequently employed (Gautam A., 2022). The traditional, well-known, straightforward, and least sophisticated feature extraction method known as the bag of words (BOW) displays the words inside a document and addresses the text as numbers. Words that frequently appear in the text are counted by BOW as features and are collected into a bag. Language structure, word placement, and word design are not factors in the BOW. For feature extraction, Bag of Phrases measures accessible keywords and uses a vocabulary of well-known words. Each word incorporates as a feature in BOW and is given equal significance (Rui W., 2016). In order to produce the feature vectors, the bag of words collects the data, builds a lexicon, and scores each document's terms. The feature frequency is represented by a value of 1 if it appears in the input data; otherwise, it is represented by a value of 0. In the case of medium-sized datasets and domain-specific circumstances, the bag of words features extraction method may outperform advanced word embedding-based features extraction methods with machine learning classifiers.

Term Frequency-Inverse Document Frequency, often known as TF-IDF, is a well-known, more precise statistical-based feature extraction technique that can determine the importance of any words in a collection of documents. Given that more often occurring words are more helpful for categorisation, the regularly occurring words in TF-IDF are given higher weight (Das B. et al., 2018). Any term's term frequency (TF) is calculated based on how many times it appears in a document relative to how many words there are overall. Any term in the documents is evaluated for importance using the inverse document frequency (IDF) method. Tomas Mikolov introduced Word2Vec, a predictive word embedding-based feature extraction technique, at Google in 2013. Word2vec is typically used to distinguish between relationships between words or things like semantic similarity, identifiable proof, thinking concept arrangement, determination inclinations, and closeness. After understanding the relationship, the Word2vec algorithm uses words from a large corpus of text data as input information and outputs a feature vector (Mikolov T., 2013). Word2Vec generates the vector representations using two distinct techniques: a continuous bag of words (CBOW) and Skip-Gram.

GloVe (Global Vectors) is a co-occurrence and count-based model that identifies co-occurring words in the corpus and generates a co-occurrence matrix for learning (Pennington D., 2014). The GloVe is easier to prepare for large information sizes and has parallel execution capabilities. FastText is a variation of Word2Vec that supports the skip-gram and CBOW methods (Continuous Word of Bag). FastText offers pre-built models that handle character-level n-grams in 157 different languages. FastText does not transcribe words directly. In order to obtain the vector representation, it first splits the terms down into a few sub-words, addresses them as n-grams of characters, and then handles them in the neural network (Joulin A., 2016). A 2-layer bi-directional deep LSTM network is used in the "ELMo" algorithm, which stands for "Embedding from Language Model," to construct vector representations of words (Peters M. E., 2018). Instead of using reference words with their vector structure, ELMo takes into account the sets in which they have been used. ELMo uses the entire sentence that contains the word in question to compute the word's embeddings. ELMo embeddings may recognise a word's context and provide distinct embeddings for a different context that is used as a replacement setting in various phrases. BERT, or "Bidirectional Encoder Representations from Transformer," is an improved prediction-based contextual embedding model that uses two distinct word vectors for a different context and makes use of deep bidirectional layers of transformer encoders. By utilising transfer, BERT creates a context-oriented relationship between any sentence's words to create the word's vector representation. BERT uses CLS, SEP, and MASK tokens for training and fine-tuning and accepts phrases as information (Devlin J.,2018).

Cyberstalking Detection

In this stage, cleaned and formatted datasets through pre-processing and feature extraction are split into training and testing datasets. Generally, researchers utilise 80% of the data from the dataset for training purposes, and 20% of data from the dataset is used for testing the machine learning classifiers. The machine learning classifiers are trained by using these training datasets. Once the classifiers are trained, they can be used for testing and classification tasks in cyberstalking detection model. Trained machine learning classifiers have the capability to predict the probability for any target class (cyberstalking or non-cyberstalking text) using the prediction or probability score based on the learning experience. After training and testing the machine learning classifiers, actual data are used in real-time to detect cyberstalking text or non-cyberstalking text. Several supervised machine learning algorithms can be used for classification tasks in cyberstalking detection model. Logistic Regression, Support Vector Machines, AdaBoost, Gradient boosting, XGBoost, Naive Bayes, Random Forest, Decision Trees, K-Nearest Neighbor are some most popular machine learning algorithms used for classification tasks in cyberstalking detection. As per available research (Devlin J., 2018) performance of support vector machines, logistic regression, and XGBoost are better than other classifiers in cyberstalking detection.

Message and Evidence Collection

During the detection of cyberstalking text in actual data in real-time, sufficient evidence against the cyberstalkers are also highly required for further legal complaints and action. The cyberstalking detection model identifies the cyberstalking text and collects all available evidence for documentation, such as the message (cyberstalking text), sender id and name (cyberstalker's profile), source of internet application, targeted victims or organisations, history of cyberstalkers, the intention of cyberstalkers, etc. Such evidence documentation is required to save into a global database and is helpful for further action and support. One of the major issues of message collection and evidence gathering is identifying cyberstalkers' actual or fake profiles. Cyberstalkers often use fake accounts on social media networks and other internet applications to target and harass the victims, which is still a challenging issue to ultimately combat the cyberstalkers using the single approach of cyberstalking detection model. In this scenario, technological support from cyberstalking detection model and service provider end (social media and other internet applications) as well as social, psychological, and law enforcement as a combined approach should be used for proper identification and combating the cyberstalking.

Performance Metrics

After detecting cyberstalking text and collecting all valuable messages and evidence documentation, the performance of the cyberstalking model is required to measure. The cyberstalking detection model's performance explains how efficient the applied cyberstalking detection model is in solving the assigned tasks. Several parameters are used to monitor and measure the performance of the cyberstalking detection model during training, testing, and application in real scenario time of the detection model, known as performance metrics. In the case of monitoring and measuring the performance of the cyberstalking detection model (binary classification), a confusion matrix is generally utilised to calculate several performance metrics parameters. The confusion matrix represents the "2x2" truth table in tabular form, containing the actual and prediction classes with the total values of true positive, true negative, false positive, and false negative. True positive represent the total correctly predicted text as cyberstalking text, while true negative show the total correctly predicted text as non-cyberstalking text. In other prediction cases, false positive refers to the total wrongly predicted text as cyberstalking text, while false negative explains the total number of wrongly predicted text as non-cyberstalking text. Several useful parameters as performance metrics, namely accuracy, precision, f-score, recall and AUC, training time, and prediction time, are widely used to measure the performance of cyberstalking detection model. Accuracy represents the number of correct predictions predicted by the cyberstalking detection model. Accuracy is calculated by the total value of true positive plus true negative divided by total prediction. Precision shows the ratio between the true positives and all the other positive values, and it is calculated by the total positive divided by the total true positive plus the total false positive. The recall represents the detection rate calculated by total true positive divided by total true positive plus total false negative. F-score shows the combined trend between recall and precision and describes the harmonic average between recall and precision.

Above cyberstalking, prevention and detection approaches based on the latest emerging technology may be helpful for the internet user. Internet users who are aware of these techniques can use the internet without any mental stress. However, if any cyberstalking event may occur, then they protect themselves and spread awareness with the help of communication technology like social media, blogs, youtube and other media.

CONCLUSION

Cyberstalking is an act of attacking or harassing anyone through a public network and is still a critical and growing issue. This chapter discussed the various cyberstalking techniques that occurred on various platforms like social media or email. Further, the consequences of cyberstalking have been discussed, which significantly impact teenagers and women. The consequences of cyberstalking have a serious impact on the mental health of the victim. The various consequences, such as physical, mental, depression, and anxiety problems, are discussed in this chapter. We also presented coping strategies such as psychological coping methods, preventive coping approaches, and detection approaches. This coping strategy may secure people from making victims of cyberstalking. Various automatic detection approaches, which are recently developed by the researcher, may also help to detect cyberstalking incidents before they happen. With the awareness of these methods, a user can use the internet without any mental stress.

REFERENCES

Acquadro Maran, D., & Begotti, T. (2019). Prevalence of cyberstalking and previous offline victimisation in a sample of Italian university students. *Social Sciences (Basel, Switzerland)*, *8*(1), 30. doi:10.3390ocsci8010030

Al-Khater, W. A., Al-Maadeed, S., Ahmed, A. A., Sadiq, A. S., & Khan, M. K. (2020). Comprehensive Review of Cybercrime Detection Techniques. *IEEE Access : Practical Innovations, Open Solutions*, *8*, 137293–137311. doi:10.1109/ACCESS.2020.3011259

Alotaibi, M., Alotaibi, B., & Razaque, A. (2021). A multichannel deep learning framework for cyberbullying detection on social media. *Electronics (Basel)*, *10*(21), 2664. doi:10.3390/electronics10212664

Asante, A., & Feng, X. (2021). Content-based technical solution for cyberstalking detection. In *2021 3rd International Conference on Computer Communication and the Internet (ICCCI)*. IEEE.

Ayo, F. E., Folorunso, O., Ibharalu, F. T., Osinuga, I. A., & Abayomi-Alli, A. (2021). A probabilistic clustering model for hate speech classification in Twitter. *Expert Systems with Applications*, *173*, 114762. doi:10.1016/j.eswa.2021.114762

Baer, M. (2020). Cyberstalking and the Internet Landscape We Have Constructed. *Virginia Journal of Law & Technology*, *154*(15), 153–227.

Begotti, T., & Acquadro Maran, D. (2019). Characteristics of cyberstalking behavior, consequences, and coping strategies: A cross-sectional study in a sample of Italian university students. *Future Internet*, *11*(5), 120. doi:10.3390/fi11050120

Begotti, T., Bollo, M., & Acquadro Maran, D. (2020). Coping strategies and anxiety and depressive symptoms in young adult victims of cyberstalking: A questionnaire survey in an Italian sample. *Future Internet*, *12*(8), 136. doi:10.3390/fi12080136

Bini, S. A. (2018). Artificial intelligence, machine learning, deep learning, and cognitive computing: What do these terms mean and how will they impact health care? *The Journal of Arthroplasty*, *33*(8), 2358–2361. doi:10.1016/j.arth.2018.02.067 PMID:29656964

Dadvar, M., de Jong, F., Ordelman, R., & Trieschnigg, D. (2012). Improved cyberbullying detection using gender information. *Proceedings of the twelfth Dutch-Belgian information retrieval workshop*, 23–25.

Das, B., & Chakraborty, S. (2018). *An improved text sentiment classification model using TF-IDF and next word negation.* arXiv preprint arXiv:1806.06407.

Derhab, A., Bouras, F. B., Muhaya, K., & Xiang. (2014). Spam trapping system: Novel security framework to fight against spam botnets. *Proc. 21st Int. Conf. Telecommun. (ICT)*, 467-471. 10.1109/ICT.2014.6845160

Devlin, J., Chang, M. W., Lee, M., & Toutanova, K. (2018). *Bert: Pre-training of deep bidirectional transformers for language understanding.* arXiv preprint arXiv:1810.04805.

Dinakar, K., Reichart, R., & Lieberman, H. (2011). Modeling the detection of textual cyberbullying. *The Social Mobile Web, 11*(02), 11–17.

Frommholz, I., & Haider, M. (2016). On Textual Analysis and Machine Learning for Cyberstalking Detection. *Datenbank-Spektrum: Zeitschrift fur Datenbanktechnologie: Organ der Fachgruppe Datenbanken der Gesellschaft fur Informatik e.V, 16*(2), 127–135. doi:10.100713222-016-0221-x PMID:29368749

Galán-GarcÍa, P., De La Puerta, J. G., Gómez, C. L., Santos, I., & Bringas, P. G. (2016). Supervised machine learning for the detection of troll profiles in Twitter social network: Application to a real case of cyberbullying. *Logic Journal of the IGPL*, 42–53.

Gautam, A. K., & Bansal, A. (2022). A Review on Cyberstalking Detection Using Machine Learning Techniques: Current Trends and Future Direction. *International Journal of Engineering Trends and Technology, 70*(3), 95–107. doi:10.14445/22315381/IJETT-V70I3P211

Gautam, A. K., & Bansal, A. (2022). Effect of features extraction techniques on cyberstalking detection using machine learning framework. *Journal of Advances in Information Technology, 13*(5).

Gautam, A. K., & Bansal, A. (2022). Performance Analysis of Supervised Machine Learning Techniques For Cyberstalking Detection In Social Media. *Journal of Theoretical and Applied Information Technology, 100*(2), 2022.

Gautam, A. K., & Bansal, A. (2023). Email-Based Cyberstalking Detection On Textual Data Using Multi-Model Soft Voting Technique Of Machine Learning Approach. *Journal of Computer Information Systems*, 1–20. doi:10.1080/088744 17.2022.2155267

Gautam, A. K., & Bansal, A. (2023). Automatic Cyberstalking Detection on Twitter in Real-Time using Hybrid Approach. *International Journal of Modern Education and Computer Science, 15*(1), 2023. doi:10.5815/ijmecs.2023.01.05

Ghasem, Z., Frommholz, I., & Maple, C. (2015). Machine learning solutions for controlling cyberbullying and cyberstalking. *International Journal of Information Security*, *6*(2), 55–64.

Hindustan Times. (2015). Available at: https://www.hindustantimes.com/mumbai/35-yr-old-first-convict-in-a-cyber-stalking-case-in-state/

Indian Express. (2020). Available at: https://indianexpress.com/article/cities/delhi/ghaziabad-man-held-for-stalking-harassing-women-6585841/

Jadhav, Y. A. (2021). Cyber Safety Against Social Media Abusing. In *International Conference on Advances in Computing and Data Sciences*. Springer. 10.1007/978-3-030-81462-5_12

Joulin, A., Grave, E., Bojanowski, P., & Mikolov, T. (2016). *Bag of tricks for efficient text classification*. arXiv preprint arXiv:1607.01759.

Kadhim, A. I. (2018). An evaluation of pre-processing techniques for text classification. *International Journal of Computer Science and Information Security*, *16*(6), 22–32.

Kamphuis, J. H., & Emmelkamp, P. M. G. (2000). stalking–a contemporary challenge for forensic and clinical psychiatry. *The British Journal of Psychiatry*, *176*(3), 206–209. doi:10.1192/bjp.176.3.206 PMID:10755065

Khader, M., & Chan, S. (2020). *Unwanted attention: a survey on cyberstalking victimisation. Psycho-Criminological Approaches to Stalking Behavior: An International Perspective. Wiley Series in the Psychology of Crime, Policing and Law*. Wiley.

Kritzinger, Bada, & Nurse. (2017). A study into the cybersecurity awareness initiatives for school learners in South Africa and the UK. In *Proc. IFIP World Conference on Information Security Education*. Springer. 10.1007/978-3-319-58553-6_10

Kumar, A., & Sachdeva. (2021). A Bi-GRU with attention and CapsNet hybrid model for cyberbullying detection on social media. *World Wide Web (Bussum)*, 1–14.

Kwan, I., Dickson, K., Richardson, M., MacDowall, W., Burchett, H., Stansfield, C., & Thomas, J. (2020). Cyberbullying and children and young people's mental health: A systematic map of systematic reviews. *Cyberpsychology, Behavior, and Social Networking*, *23*(2), 72–82. doi:10.1089/cyber.2019.0370 PMID:31977251

Melander, L. A., & Marganski, A. J. (2020). Cyber and in-person intimate partner violence victimisation: Examining maladaptive psychosocial and behavioural correlates. *Cyberpsychology (Brno)*, *14*(1). Advance online publication. doi:10.5817/CP2020-1-1

Mikolov, T., Chen, K., Corrado, G., & Dean, J. (2013). *Efficient estimation of word representations in vector space.* arXiv preprint arXiv:1301.3781.

Ministry of Law, Justice and Company Affairs (Legislative Department): Information Technology ACT (2008). https://police.py.gov.in /Information%20Technology%20 Act%202000%20-%202008%20(amendment).pdf

Mullen, P. E., Pathe, M., Purcell, R., & Stuart, G. W. (1999). Study of Stalker. *The American Journal of Psychiatry, 156*(8), 1244–1249. doi:10.1176/ajp.156.8.1244 PMID:10450267

Nahar, V., Li, X., Zhang, H. L., & Pang, C. (2014). Detecting cyberbullying in social networks using multi-agent system. *Web Intelligence and Agent Systems: An International Journal, 12*(4), 375–388. doi:10.3233/WIA-140301

Ogilvie, E. (2000). Cyberstalking. Trends and Issues in Crime and Criminal Justice. *Australian Institute of Criminology, 166*, 1.

Pennington, D., Socher, R., & Manning, C. D. (2014). Glove: Global vectors for word representation. *Proc. Conference on Empirical Methods in Natural Language Processing.*

Peters, J. F. (2017). *Foundations of computer vision: computational geometry, visual image structures and object shape detection* (Vol. 124). Springer. doi:10.1007/978-3-319-52483-2

PetersM. E.NeumannM.IyyerM.GardnerM.ClarkC.LeeK.ZettlemoyerL. (2018). *Deep contextualised word representations.* arXiv:1802.05365v2.

Prakash, R. (2019). Cyber crime: A critical study. *International Journal of Legal Developments and Allied Issues, 5*(5), 163-171. https://thelawbrigade.com/wp-content/uploads/2019/09/Rohit-prakash.pdf

Ptaszynski, M., Masui, F., Nakajima, Y., Kimura, Y., Rzepka, R., & Araki, K. (2016). *Detecting cyberbullying with morphosemantic patterns.* Paper presented at joint 8th international conference on soft computing and intelligent systems and 17th international symposium on advanced intelligent systems, Sapporo, Japan.

Raisi, E., & Huang, B. (2016). *Cyberbullying identification using participant-vocabulary consistency.* Paper presented at 2016 ICML workshop on #Data4Good: Machine learning in social good applications, New York, NY.

Rizwan, K. (2021). HarX: Real-time harassment detection tool using machine learning. In *2021 International Conference of Modern Trends in Information and Communication Technology Industry (MTICTI).* IEEE. 10.1109/MTICTI53925.2021.9664755

Rui, W., Xing, K., & Jia, Y. (2016). BOWL: Bag of word clusters text representation using word embeddings. In *Proc. International Conference on Knowledge Science, Engineering and Management*. 10.1007/978-3-319-47650-6_1

Sadiq, S., Mehmood, A., Ullah, S., Ahmad, M., Choi, G. S., & On, B.-W. (2021). Aggression detection through deep neural model on Twitter. *Future Generation Computer Systems*, *114*, 120–129. doi:10.1016/j.future.2020.07.050

Singhal, P., & Bansal, A. (2013). Improved textual cyberbullying detection using data mining. *International Journal of Information and Computation Technology*, *3*(6), 569–575.

Soundar, K. R., & Ponesakki, P. (2016). Cyberbullying Detection based on text representation. *International Journal of Engineering Science*, *6*(10), 2776–2785.

Stevens, F., Nurse, J. R., & Arief, B. (2021). Cyber stalking, cyber harassment and adult mental health: A systematic review. *Cyberpsychology, Behavior, and Social Networking*, *24*(6), 367–376. doi:10.1089/cyber.2020.0253 PMID:33181026

The National Crime Records Bureau. Crime in India. (2020). https://www. thehinducentre.com /resources/ article36608197.ece/binary/CII%202020%20 Volume%201.pdf

The Statista. (2021a). *Number of internet users in India*. Available at: https://www. statista.com/statistics/255146/number-of-internet-users-in-india/

The Statista. (2021b). *Number of social network users in India*. Available at: https:// www.statista.com/statistics/278407/number-of-social-network-users-in-india

Time of India website: Two arrested for cyberstalking. (2021). Available at: https:// timesofindia.indiatimes.com/city/hyderabad/two-arrested-for-cyber-stalking/ articleshow/ 82280780.cms

Times of India. (2021). *Beware! Cyberstalking is on the rise during the pandemic*. Available at: https://timesofindia.indiatimes.com/life-style/spotlight/beware-cyberstalking-is-on-the-rise-during-the-pandemic/articleshow/81924158.cms

Tolba, M., Ouadfel, S., & Meshoul, S. (2021). Hybrid ensemble approaches to online harassment detection in highly imbalanced data. *Expert Systems with Applications*, *175*, 114751. doi:10.1016/j.eswa.2021.114751

Truman, J. L. (2010). *Examining intimate partner stalking and use of technology in stalking victimisation* [Ph.D. thesis]. University of Central Florida Orlando, FL.

Vijayarani, & Ilamathi, & Nithya. (2015). Pre-processing techniques for text mining-an overview. *International Journal of Computer Science & Communication Networks*, *5*(1), 7–16.

Villora, B., Yubero, S., & Navarro, R. (2020). Subjective well-being among victimised university students: Comparison between cyber dating abuse and bullying victimisation. *Information Technology & People*. Advance online publication. doi:10.1108/ITP-11-2018-0535

Zainudin, N. M., Zainal, K. H., Hasbullah, N. A., Wahab, N. A., & Ramli, S. (2016). A review on cyberbullying in Malaysia from a digital forensic perspective. *Proc. International Conference on Information and Communication Technology*, 246-250. 10.1109/ICICTM.2016.7890808

Zee News website: Bulli Bai Controversy. (2021). https://zeenews.india.com/india/bulli-bai-controversy-all-you-need-to-know-about-the-app-targeting-muslim-women-on-social-media-2424831.html

Zhong, H., Li, H., Squicciarini, A. C., Rajtmajer, S. M., Griffin, C., Miller, D. J., & Caragea, C. (2016, July). Content-Driven Detection of Cyberbullying on the Instagram Social Network. *IJCAI (United States)*, *16*, 3952–3958.

Compilation of References

Abouelmehdi, K., Beni-Hessane, A., & Khaloufi, H. (2018). Big healthcare data: Preserving security and privacy. *Journal of Big Data*, *5*(1), 1. Advance online publication. doi:10.118640537-017-0110-7

Abraham, C., Chatterjee, D., & Sims, R. R. (2019). Muddling through cybersecurity: Insights from the US healthcare industry. *Business Horizons*, *62*(4), 539–548. doi:10.1016/j.bushor.2019.03.010

Acikgoz, S. U., & Diwekar, U. M. (2010). Blood glucose regulation with stochastic optimal control for insulin-dependent diabetic patients. *Chemical Engineering Science*, *65*(3), 1227–1236. doi:10.1016/j.ces.2009.09.077

Acquadro Maran, D., & Begotti, T. (2019). Prevalence of cyberstalking and previous offline victimisation in a sample of Italian university students. *Social Sciences (Basel, Switzerland)*, *8*(1), 30. doi:10.3390ocsci8010030

Adams, B. M., Banks, H. T., Kwon, H.-D., & Tran, H. T. (2004). Dynamic multidrug therapies for hiv: Optimal and sti control approaches. *Mathematical Biosciences and Engineering*, *1*(2), 223–241. doi:10.3934/mbe.2004.1.223 PMID:20369969

Agarwal, J., Christa, S. A., Pai, H., & Kumar. (2023). Machine Learning Application for News Text Classification. *13th International Conference on Cloud Computing, Data Science & Engineering (Confluence)*, 463-466. 10.1109/Confluence56041.2023.10048856

Akarca, D., Xiu, P. Y., Ebbitt, D., Mustafa, B., Al-Ramadhani, H., & Albeyatti, A. (2019, June). Blockchain secured electronic health records: patient rights, privacy and cybersecurity. In *2019 10th International Conference on Dependable Systems, Services and Technologies (DESSERT)* (pp. 108-111). IEEE.

Akbanov, M., Vassilakis, V. G., & Logothetis, M. D. (2019). Ransomware detection and mitigation using software-defined networking: The case of WannaCry. *Computers & Electrical Engineering*, *76*, 111–121. doi:10.1016/j.compeleceng.2019.03.012

Akcora, C. G., Li, Y., Gel, Y. R., & Kantarcioglu, M. (2019). *BitcoinHeist: Topological data analysis for ransomware detection on the bitcoin blockchain*. arXiv preprint arXiv:1906.07852.

Akshay Kumaar, M., Samiayya, D., Vincent, P. M. D. R., Srinivasan, K., Chang, C. Y., & Ganesh, H. (2022). A Hybrid Framework for Intrusion Detection in Healthcare Systems Using Deep Learning. *Frontiers in Public Health*, *9*, 824898. Advance online publication. doi:10.3389/fpubh.2021.824898 PMID:35096763

Alahi, A., Bierlaire, M., & Vandergheynst, P. (2014). Robust realtimepedestrians detection in urban environments with lowresolution cameras. *Transportation Research Part C, Emerging Technologies*, *39*, 113–128. doi:10.1016/j.trc.2013.11.019

Al-Haija, Q. A., McCurry, C. D., & Zein-Sabatto, S. (2020, September). Intelligent self-reliant cyber-attacks detection and classification system for IoT communication using deep convolutional neural network. In *International Networking Conference* (pp. 100-116). Springer.

Alhawi, O. M., Baldwin, J., & Dehghantanha, A. (2018). Leveraging machine learning techniques for windows ransomware network traffic detection. In *Cyber threat intelligence* (pp. 93–106). Springer. doi:10.1007/978-3-319-73951-9_5

Al-Khater, W. A., Al-Maadeed, S., Ahmed, A. A., Sadiq, A. S., & Khan, M. K. (2020). Comprehensive Review of Cybercrime Detection Techniques. *IEEE Access : Practical Innovations, Open Solutions*, *8*, 137293–137311. doi:10.1109/ACCESS.2020.3011259

Allam, Z., Dey, G., & Jones, D. S. (2020). Artificial intelligence (AI) provided early detection of the coronavirus (COVID-19) in China and will influence future urban health policy internationally. *AI*, *1*(2), 156–165. . doi:10.3390/ai1020009

Almashhadani, A. O., Kaiiali, M., Sezer, S., & O'Kane, P. (2019). A multi-classifier network-based crypto ransomware detection system: A case study of locky ransomware. *IEEE Access : Practical Innovations, Open Solutions*, *7*, 47053–47067. doi:10.1109/ACCESS.2019.2907485

Alotaibi, M., Alotaibi, B., & Razaque, A. (2021). A multichannel deep learning framework for cyberbullying detection on social media. *Electronics (Basel)*, *10*(21), 2664. doi:10.3390/electronics10212664

Alotaiby, T. N., Alshebeili, S. A., Alshawi, T., Ahmad, I., & El-Samie, F. E. A. (2014). Eeg seizure detection and prediction algorithms: A survey. *EURASIP Journal on Advances in Signal Processing*, *2014*(1), 183. doi:10.1186/1687-6180-2014-183

Alouani, D. J., Rajapaksha, R. R. P., Jani, M., Rhoads, D. D., & Sadri, N. (2021). Specificity of SARS-CoV-2 real-time PCR improved by deep learning analysis. *Journal of Clinical Microbiology*, *59*(6), e02959–e20. doi:10.1128/JCM.02959-20 PMID:33731417

Alqudaihi, K. S., Aslam, N., Khan, I. U., Almuhaideb, A. M. A. M., Alsunaidi, S. J., Ibrahim, N. M. A. R., Alhaidari, F. A., Shaikh, F. S., Alsenbel, Y. M., Alalharith, D. M., Alharthi, H. M., Alghamdi, W. M., & Alshahrani, M. S. (2021, July 15). Cough sound detection and diagnosis using artificial intelligence techniques: Challenges and opportunities. *IEEE Access : Practical Innovations, Open Solutions*, *9*, 102327–102344. doi:10.1109/ACCESS.2021.3097559 PMID:34786317

Al-rimy, B. A. S., Maarof, M. A., & Shaid, S. Z. M. (2018). Ransomware threat success factors, taxonomy, and countermeasures: A survey and research directions. *Computers & Security, 74,* 144–166. doi:10.1016/j.cose.2018.01.001

Aly, M., & Khomh, F. (2019, March 27). *Enforcing security in Internet of Things frameworks: A Systematic Literature Review.* https://www.sciencedirect.com/science/article/abs/pii/S2542660518300805

Anand Kumar, M., Abirami, N., Guru Prasad, M. S., & Mohankumar, M. (2022). Stroke Disease Prediction based on ECG Signals using Deep Learning Techniques. *2022 International Conference on Computational Intelligence and Sustainable Engineering Solutions (CISES),* 453-458. 10.1109/CISES54857.2022.9844403

Anandkumar, Agarwal, & Christa. (2023). Designing a Secure Audio / Text Based Captcha Using Neural Network. *2023 13th International Conference on Cloud Computing, Data Science & Engineering (Confluence),* 510-514. 10.1109/Confluence56041.2023.10048791

Angst, C. M., Block, E. S., D'Arcy, J., & Kelley, K. (2017). When do IT security investments matter? Accounting for the influence of institutional factors in the context of healthcare data breaches. *Management Information Systems Quarterly, 41*(3), 893–A8. doi:10.25300/MISQ/2017/41.3.10

Ardito, C., di Noia, T., di Sciascio, E., Lofù, D., Pazienza, A., & Vitulano, F. (2021). An Artificial Intelligence Cyberattack Detection System to Improve Threat Reaction in e-Health. *Italian Conference on Cybersecurity.* http://ceur-ws.org

Arevalo-Rodriguez, I., Buitrago-Garcia, D., Simancas-Racines, D., Zambrano-Achig, P., Del Campo, R., Ciapponi, A., Sued, O., Martinez-García, L., Rutjes, A. W., Low, N., Bossuyt, P. M., Perez-Molina, J. A., & Zamora, J. (2020, December 10). False-negative results of initial RT-PCR assays for COVID-19: A systematic review. *PLoS One, 15*(12), e0242958. doi:10.1371/journal.pone.0242958 PMID:33301459

Argaw, S. T., Troncoso-Pastoriza, J. R., Lacey, D., Florin, M. V., Calcavecchia, F., Anderson, D., & Flahault, A. (2020). Cybersecurity of Hospitals: Discussing the challenges and working towards mitigating the risks. *BMC Medical Informatics and Decision Making, 20*(1), 1–10. doi:10.118612911-020-01161-7 PMID:32620167

Asante, A., & Feng, X. (2021). Content-based technical solution for cyberstalking detection. In *2021 3rd International Conference on Computer Communication and the Internet (ICCCI).* IEEE.

Avijeet, B. (2022, November 30). *PCA in machine learning – Your complete guide to principal component analysis.* https://www.simplilearn.com/tutorials/machine-learning-tutorial/principal-component-analysis

Avinash, S., Naveen Kumar, H. N., Guru Prasad, M. S., Mohan Naik, R., & Parveen, G. (2023). Early Detection of Malignant Tumor in Lungs Using Feed-Forward Neural Network and K-Nearest Neighbor Classifier. *SN Computer Science, 4*(2), 195. doi:10.100742979-022-01606-y

Compilation of References

Ayo, F. E., Folorunso, O., Ibharalu, F. T., Osinuga, I. A., & Abayomi-Alli, A. (2021). A probabilistic clustering model for hate speech classification in Twitter. *Expert Systems with Applications*, *173*, 114762. doi:10.1016/j.eswa.2021.114762

Bach, L. M., Mihaljevic, B., & Zagar, M. (2018, May). Comparative analysis of blockchain consensus algorithms. In *2018 41st International Convention on Information and Communication Technology, Electronics and Microelectronics (MIPRO)* (pp. 1545-1550). IEEE. 10.23919/MIPRO.2018.8400278

Baer, M. (2020). Cyberstalking and the Internet Landscape We Have Constructed. *Virginia Journal of Law & Technology*, *154*(15), 153–227.

Begotti, T., & Acquadro Maran, D. (2019). Characteristics of cyberstalking behavior, consequences, and coping strategies: A cross-sectional study in a sample of Italian university students. *Future Internet*, *11*(5), 120. doi:10.3390/fi11050120

Begotti, T., Bollo, M., & Acquadro Maran, D. (2020). Coping strategies and anxiety and depressive symptoms in young adult victims of cyberstalking: A questionnaire survey in an Italian sample. *Future Internet*, *12*(8), 136. doi:10.3390/fi12080136

Bellman, R. E. (1983). *Mathematical methods in medicine*. World Scientific Publishing Co., Inc. doi:10.1142/0028

Ben Fekih, R., & Lahami, M. (2020, June). Application of blockchain technology in healthcare: a comprehensive study. In *International Conference on Smart Homes and Health Telematics* (pp. 268-276). Springer. 10.1007/978-3-030-51517-1_23

Bequette, B. W. (2005). A critical assessment of algorithms and challenges in the development of a closed-loop artificial pancreas. *Diabetes Technology & Therapeutics*, *7*(1), 28–47. doi:10.1089/dia.2005.7.28 PMID:15738702

Berentsen, A. (2019). *Aleksander berentsen recommends "bitcoin: a peer-to-peer electronic cash system" by Satoshi Nakamoto. In 21st Century Economics*. Springer.

Bergman, R. N., Ider, Y. Z., Bowden, C. R., & Cobelli, C. (1979). Quantitative estimation of insulin sensitivity. *American Journal of Physiology. Endocrinology and Metabolism*, *236*(6), E667. doi:10.1152/ajpendo.1979.236.6.E667 PMID:443421

Bilal, M. (2021). *Digital health: Opportunities for entrepreneurs, scientists and doctors*. https://propakistani.pk/2021/06/23/digital-health-opportunities-for-entrepreneurs-scientists-and-doctors/

Bini, S. A. (2018). Artificial intelligence, machine learning, deep learning, and cognitive computing: What do these terms mean and how will they impact health care? *The Journal of Arthroplasty*, *33*(8), 2358–2361. doi:10.1016/j.arth.2018.02.067 PMID:29656964

BlueDot. (n.d.). *Better public health surveillance for infectious diseases*. https://bluedot.global/products/explorer/

Boldyreva, A., Goyal, V., & Kumar, V. (2008, October). Identity-based encryption with efficient revocation. In *Proceedings of the 15th ACM conference on Computer and communications security* (pp. 417-426). ACM.

Bottou, L. (2012). Stochastic Gradient Descent Tricks. In Neural Networks: Tricks of the Trade (pp. 421–436). doi:10.1007/978-3-642-35289-8_25

Breiman, L. (2001, October 1). *Random Forests - Machine Learning.* https://link.springer.com/article/10.1023/A:1010933404324

Breiman, L. (2001). Random Forests. *Machine Learning, 45*(1), 5–32. doi:10.1023/A:1010933404324

Budida, D. A. M., & Mangrulkar, R. S. (2017, March). Design and implementation of smart HealthCare system using IoT. In *2017 International Conference on Innovations in Information, Embedded and Communication Systems (ICIIECS)* (pp. 1-7). IEEE. 10.1109/ICIIECS.2017.8275903

Bullock, J., Luccioni, A., Hoffman Pham, K., Sin Nga Lam, C., & Luengo-Oroz, M. (2020). Mapping the landscape of artificial intelligence applications against COVID-19. *Journal of Artificial Intelligence Research, 69*, 807–845. doi:10.1613/jair.1.12162

Burrell, D. N., Aridi, A. S., McLester, Q., Shufutinsky, A., Nobles, C., Dawson, M., & Muller, S. R. (2021). Exploring System Thinking Leadership Approaches to the Healthcare Cybersecurity Environment. *International Journal of Extreme Automation and Connectivity in Healthcare, 3*(2), 20–32. doi:10.4018/IJEACH.2021070103

Carvalho, E. D., Silva, R. R. V., Araújo, F. H. D., Rabelo, R. A. L., & de Carvalho Filho, A. O. (2021, September). An approach to the classification of COVID-19 based on CT scans using convolutional features and genetic algorithms. *Computers in Biology and Medicine, 136*, 104744. doi:10.1016/j.compbiomed.2021.104744 PMID:34388465

Chakraborty, B., & Moodie, E. (2013). *Statistical methods for dynamic treatment regimes.* Springer. doi:10.1007/978-1-4614-7428-9

Chamola, V., Hassija, V., Gupta, V., & Guizani, M. (2020). A comprehensive review of the COVID-19 pandemic and the role of IoT, drones, AI, blockchain, and 5G in managing its impact. *IEEE Access : Practical Innovations, Open Solutions, 8*, 90225–90265. doi:10.1109/ACCESS.2020.2992341

Chard, K., Bubendorfer, K., Caton, S., & Rana, O. F. (2011). Social cloud computing: A vision for socially motivated resource sharing. *IEEE Transactions on Services Computing, 5*(4), 551–563. doi:10.1109/TSC.2011.39

Chaudhary, B., & Singh, K. (2021). A Blockchain enabled location-privacy preserving scheme for vehicular ad-hoc networks. *Peer-to-Peer Networking and Applications, 14*(5), 3198–3212. doi:10.100712083-021-01079-5

Chen, J., Lim, H. W., Ling, S., Wang, H., & Nguyen, K. (2012). Revocable identity-based encryption from lattices. *Information Security and Privacy: 17th Australasian Conference, ACISP 2012, Wollongong, NSW, Australia, July 9-11, 2012 Proceedings, 17*, 390–403.

Choi, S. J., & Johnson, M. E. (2021). The relationship between cybersecurity ratings and the risk of hospital data breaches. *Journal of the American Medical Informatics Association : JAMIA, 28*(10), 2085–2092. doi:10.1093/jamia/ocab142 PMID:34338786

Cho, S., & Lee, S. (2019, January). Survey on the Application of BlockChain to IoT. In *2019 International Conference on Electronics, Information, and Communication (ICEIC)* (pp. 1-2). IEEE. 10.23919/ELINFOCOM.2019.8706369

Choucri, N. (2014). *Co-evolution of cyberspace and international relations: New challenges for the social sciences.* Academic Press.

Chu, C. K., Chow, S. S., Tzeng, W. G., Zhou, J., & Deng, R. H. (2013). Key-aggregate cryptosystem for scalable data sharing in cloud storage. *IEEE Transactions on Parallel and Distributed Systems, 25*(2), 468–477.

Chuwu, L., Chen, C.-M., Cai, Z.-X., Hsu, M. H., & Juang, W.-C. (2021). Machine learning-based detection of internet of thing attacks in healthcare environments. *IT in Industry, 9*(2).

Cimpanu, C. (2020). *Hackers preparing to launch ransomware attacks against hospitals arrested in Romania.* ZDNet. https://www. zdnet. com/ article/ hackers-preparing-to-launc h-ransomware-attacks-against-hospitals-arrested-in-romania/

Clemente, D. (2013). *Cyber security and global interdependence: what is critical?* Chatham House.

Clustering in machine learning. (n.d.a). https://www.geeksforgeeks.org/clustering-in-machine-learning/

Clustering in machine learning. (n.d.b). https://www.javatpoint.com/clustering-in-machine-learning

Cobelli, C., Renard, E., & Kovatchev, B. (2011). Artificial pancreas: Past, present, future. *Diabetes, 60*(11), 2672–2682. doi:10.2337/db11-0654 PMID:22025773

Cohen, J. P., Dao, L., Roth, K., Morrison, P., Bengio, Y., Abbasi, A. F., Shen, B., Mahsa, H. K., Ghassemi, M., Li, H., & Duong, T. Q. (2020, July). Predicting COVID-19 pneumonia severity on chest X-ray with deep learning. *Cureus, 12*(7), e9448. doi:10.7759/cureus.9448 PMID:32864270

Coronado, A. J., & Wong, T. L. (2014). Healthcare cybersecurity risk management: Keys to an effective plan. *Biomedical Instrumentation & Technology, 48*(s1), 26–30. doi:10.2345/0899-8205-48.s1.26 PMID:24848146

CrossmanL. (2020).04.20.046920. Leverging Deep Learning to stimulate coronavirus Spike proteins has the potential to predict future Zoonotic sequences. bioRxiv, 2020. https://doi.org/doi:10.1101/2020.04.20.046920

Czosseck, C., & Geers, K. (Eds.). (2009). *The virtual battlefield: perspectives on cyber warfare* (Vol. 3). IOS Press.

Dadvar, M., de Jong, F., Ordelman, R., & Trieschnigg, D. (2012). Improved cyberbullying detection using gender information. *Proceedings of the twelfth Dutch-Belgian information retrieval workshop*, 23–25.

Das, B., & Chakraborty, S. (2018). *An improved text sentiment classification model using TF-IDF and next word negation.* arXiv preprint arXiv:1806.06407.

Dasgupta, A., Sun, Y., König, I. R., Bailey-Wilson, J. E., & Malley, J. D. (2011). Brief review of regression-based and machine learning methods in genetic epidemiology: The Genetic Analysis Workshop 17 experience. *Genetic Epidemiology*, *35*(S1), S5–S11. doi:10.1002/gepi.20642 PMID:22128059

Daskalaki, E. (2013). Personalized tuning of a reinforcement learning control algorithm for glucose regulation. In *2013 35th Annual International Conference of the IEEE Engineering in Medicine and Biology Society (EMBC).* IEEE.

Daskalaki, Scarnato, Diem, & Mougiakakou. (2010). *Preliminary results of a novel approach for glucose regulation using an actor-critic learning based controller.* Academic Press.

Daskalaki, E., Diem, P., & Mougiakakou, S. G. (2013). An actor–critic based controller for glucose regulation in type 1 diabetes. *Computer Methods and Programs in Biomedicine*, *109*(2), 116–125. doi:10.1016/j.cmpb.2012.03.002 PMID:22502983

Davenport, T., & Kalakota, R. (2019). The potential for artificial intelligence in healthcare. *Future Healthcare Journal*, *6*(2), 94–102. doi:10.7861/futurehosp.6-2-94 PMID:31363513

De Aguiar, E. J., Faiçal, B. S., Krishnamachari, B., & Ueyama, J. (2020). A survey of blockchain-based strategies for healthcare. *ACM Computing Surveys*, *53*(2), 1–27. doi:10.1145/3376915

De Paula, M., Acosta, G. G., & Mart'ınez, E. C. (2015). On-line policy learning and adaptation for real-time personalization of an artificial pancreas. *Expert Systems with Applications*, *42*(4), 2234–2255. doi:10.1016/j.eswa.2014.10.038

De Paula, M., Avila, L. O., & Mart, E. C. (2015). Controlling blood glucose variability under uncertainty using reinforcement learning and gaussian processes. *Applied Soft Computing*, *35*, 310–332. doi:10.1016/j.asoc.2015.06.041

Deibert, R. J., Rohozinski, R., & Crete-Nishihata, M. (2012). Cyclones in cyberspace: Information shaping and denial in the 2008 Russia–Georgia war. *Security Dialogue*, *43*(1), 3–24. doi:10.1177/0967010611431079

Dempster, B., & Eaton-Lee, J. (2006). *Configuring IPCop Firewalls: Closing Borders with Open Source.* Packt Publishing Ltd.

Derhab, A., Bouras, F. B., Muhaya, K., & Xiang. (2014). Spam trapping system: Novel security framework to fight against spam botnets. *Proc. 21st Int. Conf. Telecommun. (ICT),* 467-471. 10.1109/ICT.2014.6845160

Devi Parameswari, C., & Mandadi, V. (2021). Public distribution system based on blockchain using solidity. In *Innovative Data Communication Technologies and Application* (pp. 175–183). Springer. doi:10.1007/978-981-15-9651-3_15

Devlin, J., Chang, M. W., Lee, M., & Toutanova, K. (2018). *Bert: Pre-training of deep bidirectional transformers for language understanding.* arXiv preprint arXiv:1810.04805.

Dhakal, S., Jaafar, F., & Zavarsky, P. (2019, January). Private blockchain network for IoT device firmware integrity verification and update. In *2019 IEEE 19th International Symposium on High Assurance Systems Engineering (HASE)* (pp. 164-170). IEEE. 10.1109/HASE.2019.00033

Dilsizian, S. E., & Siegel, E. L. (2014). Artificial intelligence in medicine and cardiac imaging: Harnessing big data and advanced computing to provide personalized medical diagnosis and treatment. *Current Cardiology Reports, 16*(1), 441. doi:10.100711886-013-0441-8 PMID:24338557

Dimitrov, D. v. (2016). Medical internet of things and big data in healthcare. In Healthcare Informatics Research (Vol. 22, Issue 3, pp. 156–163). Korean Society of Medical Informatics. doi:10.4258/hir.2016.22.3.156

Dinakar, K., Reichart, R., & Lieberman, H. (2011). Modeling the detection of textual cyberbullying. *The Social Mobile Web, 11*(02), 11–17.

Dinu, M. S. (2017). The 5th operational domain and the evolution of NATO's cyber defence concept. *Annals–Series on Military Sciences, 9*(2), 69–77.

Diro, A. A., & Chilamkurti, N. (2017, September 1). *Distributed attack detection scheme using deep learning approach for Internet of Things.* https://www.sciencedirect.com/science/article/abs/pii/S0167739X17308488

Doan, T., & Kalita, J. (2015). Selecting Machine Learning Algorithms Using Regression Models. *2015 IEEE International Conference on Data Mining Workshop (ICDMW),* 1498–1505. 10.1109/ICDMW.2015.43

Donnan, S. (2019). *Bloomberg-Are you a robot?* Bloomberg. com.

Dwivedi, S. K., Amin, R., & Vollala, S. (2020). Blockchain based secured information sharing protocol in supply chain management system with key distribution mechanism. *Journal of Information Security and Applications, 54,* 102554. doi:10.1016/j.jisa.2020.102554

Dwivedi, S. K., Roy, P., Karda, C., Agrawal, S., & Amin, R. (2021). Blockchain-based internet of things and industrial IoT: A comprehensive survey. *Security and Communication Networks, 2021,* 2021. doi:10.1155/2021/7142048

El Hajal, G., Yves, D. U. C. Q., & Börcsök, J. (2019, October). Designing and validating a cost effective safe network: application to a PACS system. In *2019 Fifth International Conference on Advances in Biomedical Engineering (ICABME)* (pp. 1-4). IEEE. 10.1109/ICABME47164.2019.8940252

Eriksson, J., & Giacomello, G. (2006). The information revolution, security, and international relations:(IR) relevant theory? *International Political Science Review*, 27(3), 221–244. doi:10.1177/0192512106064462

Ernst, D., Stan, G.-B., Goncalves, J., & Wehenkel, L. (2006). Clinical data based optimal sti strategies for hiv: a reinforcement learning approach. In *45th IEEE Conference on Decision and Control*. IEEE. 10.1109/CDC.2006.377527

Escandell-Montero, P., Mart'ınez-Mart'ınez, J. M., Mart'ın-Guerrero, J. D., Soria-Olivas, E., Vila-Frances, J., & Magdalena-Benedito, R. (2011). *Adaptive treatment of anemia on hemodialysis patients: A reinforcement learning approach. In CIDM2011*. IEEE.

Esteva, A., Robicquet, A., Ramsundar, B., Kuleshov, V., DePristo, M., Chou, K., Cui, C., Corrado, G., Thrun, S., & Dean, J. (2019). A guide to deep learning in healthcare. *Nature Medicine*, 25(1), 24–29. doi:10.103841591-018-0316-z PMID:30617335

Eun, Y. S., & Aßmann, J. S. (2016). Cyberwar: Taking stock of security and warfare in the digital age. *International Studies Perspectives*, 17(3), 343–360.

everon, D. S. (Ed.). (2012). *Cyberspace and national security: threats, opportunities, and power in a virtual world*. Georgetown University Press.

Fan, Y., Zhang, C., Liu, Z., & Qiu, Z. (2019, January 14). *Cost-Sensitive Stacked Sparse Auto-Encoder Models to Detect Striped Stem Borer Infestation on Rice Based on Hyperspectral Imaging*. https://www.sciencedirect.com/science/article/abs/pii/S0950705119300024

Feng, Q., Zhang, Y., Li, C., Dou, Z., & Wang, J. (2017, March 28). Anomaly spectrum detection in wireless communication via deep auto-encoders. *The Journal of Supercomputing*. https://link.springer.com/article/10.1007/s11227-017-2017-7

Feng, M., Valdes, G., Dixit, N., & Solberg, T. D. (2018). *Machine learning in radiation oncology: Opportunities, requirements, and needs* (Vol. 8). Frontiers in Oncology.

Foley, L., Foley, L., Hoffman, S. K., McGinley, T. G., Barney, K., Nelson, C., & Tosouni, A. (2003). *Identity theft: The aftermath 2003*. Gartner Research Group.

FoudaM.KsantiniR.ElmedanyW. (2021). A Novel Intrusion Detection System for Internet of Healthcare Things Based on Deep Subclasses Dispersion Information. TechRxiv. *Powered by IEEE*. doi:10.36227/techrxiv.19292444.v1

Frommholz, I., & Haider, M. (2016). On Textual Analysis and Machine Learning for Cyberstalking Detection. *Datenbank-Spektrum: Zeitschrift fur Datenbanktechnologie: Organ der Fachgruppe Datenbanken der Gesellschaft fur Informatik e.V*, 16(2), 127–135. doi:10.100713222-016-0221-x PMID:29368749

Fu, J. Y. L., Chong, Y. M., Sam, I. C., & Chan, Y. F. (2022). SARS-CoV-2 multiplex RT-PCR to detect variants of concern (VOCs) in Malaysia, between January to May 2021. *Journal of Virological Methods*, *301*, 114462. doi:10.1016/j.jviromet.2022.114462 PMID:35026305

Fuqaha, A., & Guizani, A. (n.d.). *Internet of Things: A Survey on Enabling Technologies, Protocols, and Applications.* https://ieeexplore.ieee.org/document/7123563

Galán-García, P., De La Puerta, J. G., Gómez, C. L., Santos, I., & Bringas, P. G. (2016). Supervised machine learning for the detection of troll profiles in Twitter social network: Application to a real case of cyberbullying. *Logic Journal of the IGPL*, 42–53.

Gautam, A. K., & Bansal, A. (2022). Effect of features extraction techniques on cyberstalking detection using machine learning framework. *Journal of Advances in Information Technology, 13*(5).

Gautam, A. K., & Bansal, A. (2022). A Review on Cyberstalking Detection Using Machine Learning Techniques: Current Trends and Future Direction. *International Journal of Engineering Trends and Technology*, *70*(3), 95–107. doi:10.14445/22315381/IJETT-V70I3P211

Gautam, A. K., & Bansal, A. (2022). Performance Analysis of Supervised Machine Learning Techniques For Cyberstalking Detection In Social Media. *Journal of Theoretical and Applied Information Technology*, *100*(2), 2022.

Gautam, A. K., & Bansal, A. (2023). Automatic Cyberstalking Detection on Twitter in Real-Time using Hybrid Approach. *International Journal of Modern Education and Computer Science*, *15*(1), 2023. doi:10.5815/ijmecs.2023.01.05

Gautam, A. K., & Bansal, A. (2023). Email-Based Cyberstalking Detection On Textual Data Using Multi-Model Soft Voting Technique Of Machine Learning Approach. *Journal of Computer Information Systems*, 1–20. doi:10.1080/08874417.2022.2155267

Gautam, T., & Jain, A. (2015). Analysis of brute force attack using TG — Dataset. *2015 SAI Intelligent Systems Conference (IntelliSys)*, 984-988. 10.1109/IntelliSys.2015.7361263

Gaweda, A. E., Muezzinoglu, M. K., Aronoff, G. R., Jacobs, A. A., Zurada, J. M., & Brier, M. E. (2005). *Reinforcement learning approach to individualization of chronic pharmacotherapy. In IJCNN'05* (Vol. 5). IEEE.

Gaži, P., Kiayias, A., & Zindros, D. (2019, May). Proof-of-stake sidechains. In *2019 IEEE Symposium on Security and Privacy (SP)* (pp. 139-156). IEEE. 10.1109/SP.2019.00040

Georgiadou, A., Mouzakitis, S., & Askounis, D. (2021). *Designing a cyber-security culture assessment survey targeting critical infrastructures during covid-19 crisis.* arXiv preprint arXiv:2102.03000.

Gervais, A., Karame, G. O., Wüst, K., Glykantzis, V., Ritzdorf, H., & Capkun, S. (2016, October). On the security and performance of proof of work blockchains. In *Proceedings of the 2016 ACM SIGSAC conference on computer and communications security* (pp. 3-16). 10.1145/2976749.2978341

Ge, Y., Tian, T., Huang, S., Wan, F., Li, J., Li, S., Wang, X., Yang, H., Hong, L., Wu, N., Yuan, E., Luo, Y., Cheng, L., Hu, C., Lei, Y., Shu, H., Feng, X., Jiang, Z., Wu, Y., ... Zeng, J. (2021). An integrative drug repositioning framework discovered a potential therapeutic agent targeting COVID-19. *Signal Transduction and Targeted Therapy*, *6*(1), 165. doi:10.103841392-021-00568-6 PMID:33895786

Ghafir, I., Prenosil, V., Hammoudeh, M., Baker, T., Jabbar, S., Khalid, S., & Jaf, S. (2018). BotDet: A system for real time botnet command and control traffic detection. *IEEE Access : Practical Innovations, Open Solutions*, *6*, 38947–38958. doi:10.1109/ACCESS.2018.2846740

Ghasem, Z., Frommholz, I., & Maple, C. (2015). Machine learning solutions for controlling cyberbullying and cyberstalking. *International Journal of Information Security*, *6*(2), 55–64.

Gifani, P., Shalbaf, A., & Vafaeezadeh, M. (2021). Automated detection of COVID-19 using ensemble of transfer learning with deep convolutional neural network based on CT scans. *International Journal of Computer Assisted Radiology and Surgery*, *16*(1), 115–123. doi:10.100711548-020-02286-w PMID:33191476

Gil-Rodríguez, J., Pérez de Rojas, J., Aranda-Laserna, P., Benavente-Fernández, A., Martos-Ruiz, M., Peregrina-Rivas, J. A., & Guirao-Arrabal, E. (2022, March). Ultrasound findings of lung ultrasonography in COVID-19: A systematic review. *European Journal of Radiology*, *148*, 110156. doi:10.1016/j.ejrad.2022.110156 PMID:35078136

Global health, infectious disease, public health education. (2021, February 19). https://www.publichealth.columbia.edu/public-health-now/news /epidemic-endemic-pandemic-what-are-differences

Goldberg, Y., & Kosorok, M. R. (2012). Q-learning with censored data. *Annals of Statistics*, *40*(1), 529. doi:10.1214/12-AOS968 PMID:22754029

Grammatikis & Moscholios. (2018, November 29). *Securing the Internet of Things: Challenges, threats, and solutions*. https://www.sciencedirect.com/science/article/abs/pii/ S2542660518301161?via%3Dihub

Green James, A. (2015). Cyber Warfare A multidisciplinary analysis. Academic Press.

Gudigar, A., Raghavendra, U., Nayak, S., Ooi, C. P., Chan, W. Y., Gangavarapu, M. R., Dharmik, C., Samanth, J., Kadri, N. A., Hasikin, K., Barua, P. D., Chakraborty, S., Ciaccio, E. J., & Acharya, U. R. (2021, December). Role of artificial intelligence in COVID-19 detection. *Sensors (Basel)*, *21*(23), 8045. doi:10.339021238045 PMID:34884045

Guez, Vincent, Avoli, & Pineau. (2008). Adaptive treatment of epilepsy via batch-mode reinforcement learning. *AAAI*, 1671–1678.

Gupta, A. (2016). Securing Cyberspace: A National Security Perspective. In Securing cyberspace: International and Asian perspectives. Institute for Defence Studies and Analyses.

Compilation of References

Guru Prasad, M. S., Agarwal, J., Christa, S., Aditya Pai, H., Kumar, M. A., & Kukreti, A. (2023). An Improved Water Body Segmentation from Satellite Images using MSAA-Net. *2023 International Conference on Machine Intelligence for GeoAnalytics and Remote Sensing (MIGARS)*, 1-4. 10.1109/MIGARS57353.2023.10064508

Guru Prasad, M. S., Naveen Kumar, H. N., Raju, K., Santhosh Kumar, D. K., & Chandrappa, S. (2023). Glaucoma Detection Using Clustering and Segmentation of the Optic Disc Region from Retinal Fundus Images. *SN Computer Science*, *4*(2), 192. doi:10.100742979-022-01592-1

Guru, P. M. S., Praveen, G. J., Dodmane, R., Sardar, T. H., Ashwitha, A., & Yeole, A. N. (2023). Brain Tumor Identification and Classification using a Novel Extraction Method based on Adapted Alexnet Architecture. *6th International Conference on Information Systems and Computer Networks (ISCON)*, 1-5. 10.1109/ISCON57294.2023.10112075

Hady, A. A., Ghubaish, A., Salman, T., Unal, D., & Jain, R. (2020). Intrusion Detection System for Healthcare Systems Using Medical and Network Data: A Comparison Study. *IEEE Access : Practical Innovations, Open Solutions*, *8*, 106576–106584. doi:10.1109/ACCESS.2020.3000421

Haq, N. F., Onik, A. R., Khan Hridoy, M. A., Rafni, M., Shah, F. M., & Farid, D. M. (2003, March 2). *Application of Machine Learning Approaches in Intrusion Detection System: A Survey.* https://thesai.org/Publications/ViewPaper?Volume=4&Issue=3&Code=IJARAI&SerialNo=2

Hasan, M., & Islam, M. M. (2019, May 20). *Attack and anomaly detection in IoT sensors in IoT sites using machine learning approaches.* https://www.sciencedirect.com/science/article/pii/S2542660519300241

Hasanova, H., Baek, U. J., Shin, M. G., Cho, K., & Kim, M. S. (2019). A survey on blockchain cybersecurity vulnerabilities and possible countermeasures. *International Journal of Network Management*, *29*(2), e2060. doi:10.1002/nem.2060

Hassani, A., & ... Reinforcement learning based control of tumor growth with chemotherapy. In *2010 International Conference on System Science and Engineering (ICSSE)*. IEEE. 10.1109/ICSSE.2010.5551776

He, Y. (2021). *Health Care Cybersecurity Challenges and Solutions Under the Climate of COVID-19: Scoping Review*. PubMed Central. www.ncbi.nlm.nih.gov/pmc/articles/PMC8059789

Hedayati, A. (2012). An analysis of identity theft: Motives, related frauds, techniques and prevention. *Journal of Law and Conflict Resolution*, *4*(1), 1–12.

Heidari, M., Mirniaharikandehei, S., Khuzani, A. Z., Danala, G., Qiu, Y., & Zheng, B. (2020). Improving the performance of CNN to predict the likelihood of COVID-19 using chest X-ray images with preprocessing algorithms. *International Journal of Medical Informatics*, *144*, 104284. doi:10.1016/j.ijmedinf.2020.104284 PMID:32992136

Heilweil, R. (n.d.). *How AI is battling the coronavirus Outbreak*. Available online: https://www.com/recode/2020/1/28/21110902/artificial-intelligence-ai-coronavirus-wuhan

Hemdan & Karar. (2020). *COVIDX-net: A framework of deep learning classifiers to diagnose COVID-19*. https://arxiv.org/abs/2003.11055

He, Y., Aliyu, A., Evans, M., & Luo, C. (2021). Health care cybersecurity challenges and solutions under the climate of COVID-19: Scoping review. *Journal of Medical Internet Research*, *23*(4), e21747. doi:10.2196/21747 PMID:33764885

Hindustan Times. (2015). Available at: https://www.hindustantimes.com/mumbai/35-yr-old-first-convict-in-a-cyber-stalking-case-in-state/

Hirano, M., & Kobayashi, R. (2019, October). Machine learning based ransomware detection using storage access patterns obtained from live-forensic hypervisor. In *2019 sixth international conference on internet of things: Systems, Management and security (IOTSMS)* (pp. 1-6). IEEE. 10.1109/IOTSMS48152.2019.8939214

Hireche, R., Mansouri, H., & Pathan, A.-S. K. (2022). Security and Privacy Management in Internet of Medical Things (IoMT): A Synthesis. *Journal of Cybersecurity and Privacy*, *2*(3), 640–661. doi:10.3390/jcp2030033

Hou, H. (2017, July). The application of blockchain technology in E-government in China. In *2017 26th International Conference on Computer Communication and Networks (ICCCN)* (pp. 1-4). IEEE. 10.1109/ICCCN.2017.8038519

Hovorka, R., Canonico, V., Chassin, L. J., Haueter, U., Massi-Benedetti, M., Federici, M. O., Pieber, T. R., Schaller, H. C., Schaupp, L., Vering, T., & Wilinska, M. E. (2004). Nonlinear model predictive control of glucose concentration in subjects with type 1 diabetes. *Physiological Measurement*, *25*(4), 905–920. doi:10.1088/0967-3334/25/4/010 PMID:15382830

How are AI-based solutions being used to combat COVID-19? (n.d.). http://indiaai.gov.in/article/how-are-ai-based-solutions-being-used-to-combat-covid-19

How India fights COVID with artificial intelligence. (2021). https://analyticsindiamag.com/how-india-fights-covid-with-artificial-intelligence/

Huang, X., Liu, J. K., Tang, S., Xiang, Y., Liang, K., Xu, L., & Zhou, J. (2014). Cost-effective authentic and anonymous data sharing with forward security. *IEEE Transactions on Computers*, *64*(4), 971–983. doi:10.1109/TC.2014.2315619

Hu, C., Lovejoy, W. S., & Shafer, S. L. (1994). Comparison of some control strategies for three-compartment pk/pd models. *Journal of Pharmacokinetics and Biopharmaceutics*, *22*(6), 525–550. doi:10.1007/BF02353793 PMID:7473080

Humphrey. (2017). *Using reinforcement learning to personalize dosing strategies in a simulated cancer trial with high dimensional data*. Academic Press.

Hussain, F., Abbas, S. G., Shah, G. A., Pires, I. M., Fayyaz, U. U., Shahzad, F., Garcia, N. M., & Zdravevski, E. (2021). A framework for malicious traffic detection in iot healthcare environment. *Sensors (Basel)*, *21*(9), 3025. Advance online publication. doi:10.339021093025 PMID:33925813

Compilation of References

Indian Express. (2020). Available at: https://indianexpress.com/article/cities/delhi/ ghaziabad-ma n-held-for-stalking-harassing-women-6585841/

Introduction to support vector machines (SVM). (n.d.). https://www.geeksforgeeks.org/ introduction-to-support-vector-machines-svm/

Iwendi, C., Khan, S., Anajemba, J. H., Mittal, M., Alenezi, M., & Alazab, M. (2020, April 30). l *The Use of Ensemble Models for Multiple Class and Binary Class Classification for Improving Intrusion Detection Systems.* https://www.mdpi.com/1424-8220/20/9/2559

Jabbar, M. A. (2021). Breast cancer data classification using ensemble machine learning. *Engineering and Applied Science Research*, *48*(1), 65–72.

Jadhav, Y. A. (2021). Cyber Safety Against Social Media Abusing. In *International Conference on Advances in Computing and Data Sciences.* Springer. 10.1007/978-3-030-81462-5_12

Jain, A., Singh, T., & Sharma, S. K. (2021). Security as a solution: An intrusion detection system using a neural network for IoT enabled healthcare ecosystem. *Interdisciplinary Journal of Information, Knowledge, and Management*, *16*, 331–369. doi:10.28945/4838

Jalalimanesh, A., Haghighi, H. S., Ahmadi, A., Hejazian, H., & Soltani, M. (2017). Multi-objective optimization of radiotherapy: Distributed q-learning and agent-based simulation. *Journal of Experimental & Theoretical Artificial Intelligence*, *29*(5), 1–16. doi:10.1080/09528 13X.2017.1292319

Jalalimanesh, A., Haghighi, H. S., Ahmadi, A., & Soltani, M. (2017). Simulation-based optimization of radiotherapy: Agent-based modeling and reinforcement learning. *Mathematics and Computers in Simulation*, *133*, 235–248. doi:10.1016/j.matcom.2016.05.008

Javaid, M., Haleem, A., Pratap Singh, R., Suman, R., & Rab, S. (2022). Significance of machine learning in healthcare: Features, pillars and applications. *International Journal of Intelligent Networks*, *3*, 58–73. doi:10.1016/j.ijin.2022.05.002

Jelliffe, R. W., Buell, J., Kalaba, R., Sridhar, R., & Rockwell, R. (1970). A computer program for digitalis dosage regimens. *Mathematical Biosciences*, *9*, 179–193. doi:10.1016/0025-5564(70)90103-3

Johnson, A. E., Ghassemi, M. M., Nemati, S., Niehaus, K. E., Clifton, D. A., & Clifford, G. D. (2016). Machine learning and decision support in critical care. *Proceedings of the IEEE*, *104*(2), 444–466. doi:10.1109/JPROC.2015.2501978 PMID:27765959

Joulin, A., Grave, E., Bojanowski, P., & Mikolov, T. (2016). *Bag of tricks for efficient text classification.* arXiv preprint arXiv:1607.01759.

Kadhim, A. I. (2018). An evaluation of pre-processing techniques for text classification. *International Journal of Computer Science and Information Security*, *16*(6), 22–32.

Kajabad, E. N., & Ivanov, S. V. (2019). People detection and finding attractive areas by the use of movement detection analysis and deep learning approach. *Procedia Computer Science*, *156*, 327–337. doi:10.1016/j.procs.2019.08.209

Kamphuis, J. H., & Emmelkamp, P. M. G. (2000). stalking–a contemporary challenge for forensic and clinical psychiatry. *The British Journal of Psychiatry*, *176*(3), 206–209. doi:10.1192/bjp.176.3.206 PMID:10755065

Karapapas, C., Pittaras, I., Fotiou, N., & Polyzos, G. C. (2020, May). Ransomware as a service using smart contracts and IPFS. In *2020 IEEE International Conference on Blockchain and Cryptocurrency (ICBC)* (pp. 1-5). IEEE. 10.1109/ICBC48266.2020.9169451

Karmakar, K. K., Varadharajan, V., Tupakula, U., Nepal, S., & Thapa, C. (2020). Towards a Security Enhanced Virtualised Network Infrastructure for Internet of Medical Things (IoMT). *IEEE International Conference on Network Softwarization (NetSoft)*, 257–261. 10.1109/NetSoft48620.2020.9165387

Kashani, M. H., Madanipour, M., Nikravan, M., Asghari, P., & Mahdipour, E. (2021). A systematic review of IoT in healthcare: Applications, techniques, and trends. *Journal of Network and Computer Applications*, *192*, 103164. doi:10.1016/j.jnca.2021.103164

Kaur, G., Tomar, P., & Singh, P. (2018). Design of cloud-based green IoT architecture for smart cities. In *Internet of things and big data analytics toward next-generation intelligence* (pp. 315–333). Springer., doi:10.1007/978-3-319-60435-0_13

Kawaguchi. (2016). Bounded optimal exploration in mdp. *AAAI*, 1758–1764.

Kayode Saheed, Y., Idris Abiodun, A., Misra, S., Kristiansen Holone, M., & Colomo-Palacios, R. (2022). A machine learning-based intrusion detection for detecting internet of things network attacks. *Alexandria Engineering Journal*, *61*(12), 9395–9409. doi:10.1016/j.aej.2022.02.063

Kernel, S. V. M. (n.d.). *Functions – 'Coz your SVM knowledge is incomplete without it*. https://techvidvan.com/tutorials/svm-kernel-functions/

Keshavarzi Arshadi, A., Webb, J., Salem, M., Cruz, E., Calad-Thomson, S., Ghadirian, N., Collins, J., Diez-Cecilia, E., Kelly, B., Goodarzi, H., & Yuan, J. S. (2020, August 18). Artificial intelligence for COVID-19 drug discovery and vaccine development. *Frontiers in Artificial Intelligence*, *3*, 65. doi:10.3389/frai.2020.00065 PMID:33733182

Khader, M., & Chan, S. (2020). *Unwanted attention: a survey on cyberstalking victimisation. Psycho-Criminological Approaches to Stalking Behavior: An International Perspective. Wiley Series in the Psychology of Crime, Policing and Law*. Wiley.

Khan, S. H., Hayat, M., Bennamoun, M., & Sohel, F. A. (2018, August 1). *Cost-Sensitive Learning of Deep Feature Representations From Imbalanced Data*. https://pubmed.ncbi.nlm.nih.gov/28829320/

Khan, A. G., Zahid, A. H., Hussain, M., Farooq, M., Riaz, U., & Alam, T. M. (2019, November). A journey of WEB and Blockchain towards the Industry 4.0: An Overview. In *2019 International Conference on Innovative Computing (ICIC)* (pp. 1-7). IEEE. 10.1109/ICIC48496.2019.8966700

Khanna, V. V., Chadaga, K., Sampathila, N., Prabhu, S., Chadaga, R., & Umakanth, S. (2022). Diagnosing COVID-19 using artificial intelligence: A comprehensive review. *Network Modeling and Analysis in Health Informatics and Bioinformatics, 11*(1), 25. doi:10.100713721-022-00367-1

Kirubasri, G., Sankar, S., & Guru Prasad, M. S. (2023). *LQETA-RP: link quality based energy and trust aware routing protocol for wireless multimedia sensor networks.* Int J Syst Assur Eng Manag. doi:10.100713198-023-01873-9

K-nearest neighbor (KNN) algorithm for machine learning. (n.d.). https://www.javatpoint.com/k-nearest-neighbor-algorithm-for-machine-learning

Kodali, R. K., Swamy, G., & Lakshmi, B. (2015, December). An implementation of IoT for healthcare. In 2015 IEEE Recent Advances in Intelligent Computational Systems (RAICS) (pp. 411-416). IEEE. doi:10.1109/RAICS.2015.7488451

Koser, M., & Thaver, M. (2020). *In 5 days, over 40,000 Chinese Searches for Vulnerabilities in Indian Cyber space.* https://epaper.indianexpress.com/c/52967213

Kostyuk, N., & Zhukov, Y. M. (2019). Invisible digital front: Can cyber attacks shape battlefield events? *The Journal of Conflict Resolution, 63*(2), 317–347. doi:10.1177/0022002717737138

Kouhizadeh, M., & Sarkis, J. (2018). Blockchain practices, potentials, and perspectives in greening supply chains. *Sustainability (Basel), 10*(10), 3652. doi:10.3390u10103652

Kovatchev, Breton, Dalla Man, & Cobelli. (2009). *In silico preclinical trials: a proof of concept in closed-loop control of type 1 diabetes.* Academic Press.

Kozik, R., Choraś, M., Ficco, M., & Palmieri, F. (2022, January 1). *Semantic Scholar is a scalable, distributed machine learning approach for attack detection in edge computing environments.* https://www.semanticscholar.org/paper/A-scalable-distributed-machine-learning-approach-in-Kozik-Chora%C5%9B/eb9d71f3214e793a579d6c3cea9240f882f65d14

Kritzinger, Bada, & Nurse. (2017). A study into the cybersecurity awareness initiatives for school learners in South Africa and the UK. In *Proc. IFIP World Conference on Information Security Education.* Springer. 10.1007/978-3-319-58553-6_10

Kruse, C. S., Frederick, B., Jacobson, T., & Monticone, D. K. (2017). Cybersecurity in healthcare: A systematic review of modern threats and trends. *Technology and Health Care, 25*(1), 1–10. doi:10.3233/THC-161263 PMID:27689562

Kumaar, M. A., Samiayya, D., Durai Raj Vincent, P. M., Srinivasan, K., Chang, C.-Y., & Ganesh, H. (2001, January 1). A Hybrid Framework for Intrusion Detection in Healthcare Systems Using Deep Learning. *Frontiers.* https://www.frontiersin.org/articles/10.3389/fpubh.2021.824898/full

Kumar, A., & Sachdeva. (2021). A Bi-GRU with attention and CapsNet hybrid model for cyberbullying detection on social media. *World Wide Web (Bussum)*, 1–14.

Kumar, M. A., Pai, A. H., Agarwal, J., Christa, S., Prasad, G. M. S., & Saifi, S. (2023). *Deep Learning Model to Defend against Covert Channel Attacks in the SDN Networks. In Advanced Computing and Communication Technologies for High Performance Applications*. ACCTHPA. doi:10.1109/ACCTHPA57160.2023.10083336

Kumar, P., & Lee, H.-J. (2011). Security Issues in Healthcare Applications Using Wireless Medical Sensor Networks: A Survey. *Sensors (Basel)*, *12*(1), 55–91. doi:10.3390120100055 PMID:22368458

Kumar, R., Zhang, X., Wang, W., Khan, R. U., Kumar, J., & Sharif, A. (2019). A multimodal malware detection technique for Android IoT devices using various features. *IEEE Access : Practical Innovations, Open Solutions*, *7*, 64411–64430. doi:10.1109/ACCESS.2019.2916886

Kwan, I., Dickson, K., Richardson, M., MacDowall, W., Burchett, H., Stansfield, C., & Thomas, J. (2020). Cyberbullying and children and young people's mental health: A systematic map of systematic reviews. *Cyberpsychology, Behavior, and Social Networking*, *23*(2), 72–82. doi:10.1089/cyber.2019.0370 PMID:31977251

Laber, E. B., Linn, K. A., & Stefanski, L. A. (2014). Interactive model building for q-learning. *Biometrika*, *101*(4), 831–847. doi:10.1093/biomet/asu043 PMID:25541562

Laguarta, J., Hueto, F., & Subirana, B. (2020). COVID-19 artificial intelligence diagnosis using only cough recordings. *IEEE Open Journal of Engineering in Medicine and Biology*, *1*, 275–281. doi:10.1109/OJEMB.2020.3026928 PMID:34812418

Le, Y., Wang, Z. J., Quan, Z., He, J., & Yao, B. (2018, July). ACV-tree: A New Method for Sentence Similarity Modeling. IJCAI, 4137-4143.

Lee, Y., Kim, Y. S., Lee, D. I., Jeong, S., Kang, G. H., Jang, Y. S., Kim, W., Choi, H. Y., Kim, J. G., & Choi, S. H. (2022). The application of a deep learning system developed to reduce the time for RT-PCR in COVID-19 detection. *Scientific Reports*, *12*(1), 1234. doi:10.103841598-022-05069-2 PMID:35075153

Lesson 1: Introduction to epidemiology. (n.d.). https://www.cdc.gov/csels/dsepd/ss1978/lesson1/section11.html

Liang, K., Liu, J. K., Wong, D. S., & Susilo, W. (2014). An efficient cloud-based revocable identity-based proxy re-encryption scheme for public clouds data sharing. *Computer Security-ESORICS 2014: 19th European Symposium on Research in Computer Security, Wroclaw, Poland, September 7-11, 2014 Proceedings*, *19*(Part I), 257–272.

Libert, B., & Vergnaud, D. (2009). Adaptive-ID secure revocable identity-based encryption. In *Topics in Cryptology–CT-RSA 2009: The Cryptographers' Track at the RSA Conference 2009, San Francisco, CA, USA, April 20-24, 2009. Proceedings* (pp. 1-15). Springer Berlin Heidelberg. 10.1007/978-3-642-00862-7_1

Compilation of References

Li, M., Zhang, Z., Cao, W., Liu, Y., Du, B., Chen, C., Liu, Q., Uddin, M. N., Jiang, S., Chen, C., Zhang, Y., & Wang, X. (2020). Identifying novel factors associated with COVID-19 transmission and fatality using the machine learning approach. *The Science of the Total Environment*, *10*(764), 142810. doi:10.1016/j.scitotenv.142810 PMID:33097268

LittmanM. L. (2015). Reinforcement learning improves behaviour from evaluative feedback. *Nature, 521*(7553), 445.

Liu, G., Carter, B., Bricken, T., Jain, S., Viard, M., Carrington, M., & Gifford, D. K. (2020). Computationally optimized SARS-CoV-2 MHC Class I and II Vaccine Formulations Predicted to Target Human Haplotype Distributions. *Cell Systems*, *11*(2), 131–144.e6. doi:10.1016/j.cels.2020.06.009 PMID:32721383

Liu, G., Carter, B., & Gifford, D. K. (2021). Predicted gaps for SARS-CoV-2 subunit vaccines and their augmentation by compact peptide sets. *Cell Systems*, *12*(1), 102–107.e4. doi:10.1016/j.cels.2020.11.010 PMID:33321075

Liu, M., Wu, K., & Xu, J. J. (2019). How will blockchain technology impact auditing and accounting: Permissionless versus permissioned blockchain. *Current Issues in Auditing*, *13*(2), A19–A29. doi:10.2308/ciia-52540

Li, X., Yu, J., Zhang, Z., Ren, J., Peluffo, A. E., Zhang, W., Zhao, Y., Wu, J., Yan, K., Cohen, D., & Wang, W. (2021). Network bioinformatics analysis provides insight into drug repurposing for COVID-19. *Medicine in Drug Discovery*, *10*, 100090. doi:10.1016/j.medidd.2021.100090 PMID:33817623

Lockl, J., Schlatt, V., Schweizer, A., Urbach, N., & Harth, N. (2020). Toward trust in Internet of Things ecosystems: Design principles for blockchain-based IoT applications. *IEEE Transactions on Engineering Management*, *67*(4), 1256–1270. doi:10.1109/TEM.2020.2978014

Lopez-Martin, M., Carro, B., Sanchez-Esguevillas, A., & Lloret, J. (2017, August 26). *Conditional Variational Autoencoder for Prediction and Feature Recovery Applied to Intrusion Detection in IoT*. https://www.mdpi.com/1424-8220/17/9/1967

Madaan, L., Kumar, A., & Bhushan, B. (2020, April). Working principle, application areas and challenges for blockchain technology. In *2020 IEEE 9th international conference on communication systems and network technologies (CSNT)* (pp. 254-259). IEEE. 10.1109/CSNT48778.2020.9115794

Maher, B. S. (2011). Some thoughts on health care exchanges: Choice, defaults, and the unconnected. *Connecticut Law Review*, *44*, 1099.

Manfredi, M., Vezzani, R., Calderara, S., & Cucchiara, R. (2014). Detection of static groups and crowds gathered in open spaces by texture classification. *Pattern Recognition Letters*, *44*, 39–48. doi:10.1016/j.patrec.2013.11.001

Maniath, S., Ashok, A., Poornachandran, P., Sujadevi, V. G., AU, P. S., & Jan, S. (2017, October). Deep learning LSTM based ransomware detection. In *2017 Recent Developments in Control, Automation & Power Engineering (RDCAPE)* (pp. 442-446). IEEE.

Mankodiya, H., Palkhiwala, P., Gupta, R., Jadav, N. K., Tanwar, S., Neagu, B.-C., Grigoras, G., Alqahtani, F., & Shehata, A. M. (2022). A real-time CrowdsensingFramework for potential COVID-19 carrier detection using wearable sensors. *Mathematics*, *10*(16), 2927. doi:10.3390/math10162927

Martins, N. (n.d.). *How healthcare is using big data and AI to cure disease.* https://www.forbes.com/sites/nicolemartin1/2019/08/30/how-healthcare-is-using-big-data-and-ai-to-cure-disease/#7ebe957645cf

Matsuda, S., & Yoshimura, H. (2022). Personal identification with artificial intelligence under COVID-19 crisis: A scoping review. *Systematic Reviews*, *11*(1), 7. doi:10.118613643-021-01879-z PMID:34991695

Melander, L. A., & Marganski, A. J. (2020). Cyber and in-person intimate partner violence victimisation: Examining maladaptive psychosocial and behavioural correlates. *Cyberpsychology (Brno)*, *14*(1). Advance online publication. doi:10.5817/CP2020-1-1

Meng, T., Zhao, Y., Wolter, K., & Xu, C. Z. (2021). On consortium blockchain consistency: A queueing network model approach. *IEEE Transactions on Parallel and Distributed Systems*, *32*(6), 1369–1382. doi:10.1109/TPDS.2021.3049915

Mikolov, T., Chen, K., Corrado, G., & Dean, J. (2013). *Efficient estimation of word representations in vector space.* arXiv preprint arXiv:1301.3781.

Ministry of Law, Justice and Company Affairs (Legislative Department): Information Technology ACT (2008). https://police.py.gov.in /Information%20Technology%20Act%202000%20-%20 2008%20(amendment).pdf

Mitchell, R., & Chen, I.-R. (2014, April 1). A survey of intrusion detection techniques for cyber-physical systems. *ACM Computing Surveys.* https://dl.acm.org/doi/10.1145/2542049

Mnih, V., Kavukcuoglu, K., Silver, D., Rusu, A. A., Veness, J., Bellemare, M. G., Graves, A., Riedmiller, M., Fidjeland, A. K., Ostrovski, G., Petersen, S., Beattie, C., Sadik, A., Antonoglou, I., King, H., Kumaran, D., Wierstra, D., Legg, S., & Hassabis, D. (2015). Human-level control through deep reinforcement learning. *Nature*, *518*(7540), 529–533. doi:10.1038/nature14236 PMID:25719670

Mohammed, R., Alubady, R., & Sherbaz, A. (2021). Utilizing blockchain technology for IoT-based healthcare systems. *Journal of Physics: Conference Series*, *1818*(1), 012111. doi:10.1088/1742-6596/1818/1/012111

Mohurle, S., & Patil, M. (2017). A brief study of wannacry threat: Ransomware attack 2017. *International Journal of Advanced Research in Computer Science*, *8*(5), 1938–1940.

Mucherino, A., Papajorgji, P. J., & Pardalos, P. M. (2009). k-Nearest Neighbor Classification. In Springer Optimization and Its Applications (pp. 83–106). doi:10.1007/978-0-387-88615-2_4

Mujeye, S. (2022). Ransomware: To Pay or Not to Pay? The results of what IT professionals recommend. In *2022 The 5th International Conference on Software Engineering and Information Management (ICSIM)* (pp. 76-81). Academic Press.

Mukherjee, H., Ghosh, S., Dhar, A., Obaidullah, S. M., Santosh, K. C., & Roy, K. (2021). Deep neural network to detect COVID-19: One architecture for both CT Scans and Chest X-rays. *Applied Intelligence*, *51*(5), 2777–2789. doi:10.100710489-020-01943-6 PMID:34764562

Mullen, P. E., Pathe, M., Purcell, R., & Stuart, G. W. (1999). Study of Stalker. *The American Journal of Psychiatry*, *156*(8), 1244–1249. doi:10.1176/ajp.156.8.1244 PMID:10450267

Murphy, S. A., Oslin, D. W., Rush, A. J., & Zhu, J. (2007). Methodological challenges in constructing effective treatment sequences for chronic psychiatric disorders. *Neuropsychopharmacology*, *32*(2), 257–262. doi:10.1038j.npp.1301241 PMID:17091129

N. H. R. G. P. M., S. B., Jain, & Anadkumar. (2022). E-Voting System Using Blockchain Technology. *4th International Conference on Advances in Computing, Communication Control and Networking (ICAC3N)*, 2106-2111. 10.1109/ICAC3N56670.2022.10074164

Nahar, V., Li, X., Zhang, H. L., & Pang, C. (2014). Detecting cyberbullying in social networks using multi-agent system. *Web Intelligence and Agent Systems: An International Journal*, *12*(4), 375–388. doi:10.3233/WIA-140301

Naïve Bayes classifier algorithm. (n.d.). https://www.javatpoint.com/machine-learning-naive-bayes-classifier

Narin, A., Kaya, C., & Pamuk, Z. (2021). Automatic detection of coronavirus disease (COVID-19) using X-ray images and deep convolutional neural networks. *Pattern Analysis & Applications*, *24*(3), 1207–1220. doi:10.100710044-021-00984-y PMID:33994847

Nayak, S. R., Nayak, D. R., Sinha, U., Arora, V., & Pachori, R. B. (2021, February). Application of deep learning techniques for detection of COVID-19 cases using chest X-ray images: A comprehensive study. *Biomedical Signal Processing and Control*, *64*, 102365. doi:10.1016/j.bspc.2020.102365 PMID:33230398

Negi, H. S., Dimri, S. C., Kumar, B., & Singh, A. (2022). Crop Prediction Based on Soil Properties using Machine Learning for Smart Farming. *2022 International Conference on Computational Intelligence and Sustainable Engineering Solutions (CISES)*, 366–370. 10.1109/CISES54857.2022.9844274

Newaz, A. I., Sikder, A. K., Babun, L., & Uluagac, A. S. (2020). HEKA: A Novel Intrusion Detection System for Attacks to Personal Medical Devices. *2020 IEEE Conference on Communications and Network Security (CNS)*, 1–9. 10.1109/CNS48642.2020.9162311

Ngo, P. D., Wei, S., Holubová, A., Muzik, J., & Godtliebsen, F. (2018). *Control of blood glucose for type-1 diabetes by using reinforcement learning with feedforward algorithm* (Vol. 2018). Computational and Mathematical Methods in Medicine.

Ngo, P. D., Wei, S., Holubova, A., Muzik, J., & Godtliebsen, F. (2018). Reinforcement-learning optimal control for type-1 diabetes. In *2018 IEEE EMBS International Conference on Biomedical & Health Informatics (BHI)*. IEEE. 10.1109/BHI.2018.8333436

Nguyen, P. Q., Soenksen, L. R., Donghia, N. M., Angenent-Mari, N. M., de Puig, H., Huang, A., Lee, R., Slomovic, S., Galbersanini, T., Lansberry, G., Sallum, H. M., Zhao, E. M., Niemi, J. B., & Collins, J. J. (2021). Wearable materials with embedded synthetic biology sensors for biomolecule detection. *Nature Biotechnology, 39*(11), 1366–1374. doi:10.103841587-021-00950-3 PMID:34183860

Nicolas Mazzucchi, A. D. (2019). *Web wars: Preparing for the next Cyber Crisis – new perspectives on shared security: NATO's next 70 Years, Carnegie Europe*. Available at: https://carnegieeurope.eu/2019/11/28/web-wars-preparing-for-next-cyber-crisis-pub-80420

Nijim, Hisham, Albataineh, Khan, & Rao. (n.d.). *FastDetict: A Data Mining Engine for Predicting and Preventing DDoS Attacks*. Retrieved September 2, 2022, from https://chem.ckcest.cn/Proceeding/Details?id=77324

Norman, M. D., Karavas, Y. G., & Reed, H. (2018, July). The emergence of trust and value in public blockchain networks. In *IX International Conference on Complex Systems* (p. 22). Academic Press.

Nye, J. S. Jr. (2010). *Cyber power*. Harvard Univ Cambridge MA Belfer Center for Science and International Affairs.

Ogilvie, E. (2000). Cyberstalking. Trends and Issues in Crime and Criminal Justice. *Australian Institute of Criminology, 166*, 1.

Olivier, B., Yonghua, Y., & Erol, G. (2018, July 30). *Deep Learning with Dense Random Neural Network for Detecting Attacks against IoT-connected Home Environments*. https://www.sciencedirect.com/science/article/pii/S1877050918311487

Ong, E., Wong, M. U., Huffman, A., & He, Y. (2020). COVID-19 coronavirus vaccine design using reverse vaccinology and machine learning. *Frontiers in Immunology, 11*, 1581. doi:10.3389/fimmu.2020.01581 PMID:32719684

Organization, W. H. (2005). *Preventing chronic diseases: a vital investment*. World Health Organization.

Ormoneit, D., & Sen, S. (2013). Kernel-based reinforcement learning. *Machine Learning, 49*(2-3), 161–178. PMID:23845276

Oso, A. A., Adefurin, A., Benneman, M. M., Oso, O. O., Taiwo, M. A., Adebiyi, O. O., & Oluwole, O. (2019). Health insurance status affects hypertension control in a hospital based internal medicine clinic. *International Journal of Cardiology. Hypertension*, *1*, 100003. doi:10.1016/j.ijchy.2019.100003 PMID:33447737

Özbilge, E., Sanlidag, T., Ozbilge, E., & Baddal, B. (2022). Artificial intelligence-assisted RT-PCR detection model for rapid and reliable diagnosis of COVID-19. *Applied Sciences (Basel, Switzerland)*, *12*(19), 9908. doi:10.3390/app12199908

Padmanabhan, R., Meskin, N., & Haddad, W. M. (2017). Reinforcement learning-based control of drug dosing for cancer chemotherapy treatment. *Mathematical Biosciences*, *293*, 11–20. doi:10.1016/j.mbs.2017.08.004 PMID:28822813

Pajouh, H.H., Javidan, R., Khayami, R., Ali, D., & K, C. K. R. (n.d.). *A Two-Layer Dimension Reduction and Two-Tier Classification Model for Anomaly-Based Intrusion Detection in IoT Backbone Networks*. https://ieeexplore.ieee.org/document/7762123

Pande, S., & Khamparia, A. (2021, June 25). *An intrusion detection system for healthcare system using machine and deep learning*. Emerald Insight. https://www.emerald.com/insight/content/doi/10.1108/WJE-04-2021-0204/full/html

Panwar, H., Gupta, P. K., Siddiqui, M. K., Morales-Menendez, R., & Singh, V. (2020). Application of deep learning for fast detection of COVID-19 in X-rays using nCOVnet. *Chaos, Solitons, and Fractals*, *138*, 109944. doi:10.1016/j.chaos.2020.109944 PMID:32536759

Parbhoo, S. (2014). *A reinforcement learning design for HIV clinical trials* [Ph.D. dissertation].

Patel, V. L., Shortliffe, E. H., Stefanelli, M., Szolovits, P., Berthold, M. R., Bellazzi, R., & Abu-Hanna, A. (2009). The coming of age of artificial intelligence in medicine. *Artificial Intelligence in Medicine*, *46*(1), 5–17. doi:10.1016/j.artmed.2008.07.017 PMID:18790621

Pazis & Parr. (2013). Pac optimal exploration in continuous space Markov decision processes. *AAAI*.

Pecoraro, V., Negro, A., Pirotti, T., & Trenti, T. (2022, February). Estimate false-negative RT-PCR rates for SARS-CoV-2. A systematic review and meta-analysis. *European Journal of Clinical Investigation*, *52*(2), e13706. doi:10.1111/eci.13706 PMID:34741305

Peng, L., Feng, W., Yan, Z., Li, Y., Zhou, X., & Shimizu, S. (2021). Privacy preservation in permissionless blockchain: A survey. *Digital Communications and Networks*, *7*(3), 295–307. doi:10.1016/j.dcan.2020.05.008

Pennington, D., Socher, R., & Manning, C. D. (2014). Glove: Global vectors for word representation. *Proc. Conference on Empirical Methods in Natural Language Processing*.

Pérez-Ortiz, M., Jiménez-Fernández, S., Gutiérrez, P. A., Alexandre, E., Hervás-Martínez, C., & Salcedo-Sanz, S. (2016). A review of classification problems and algorithms in renewable energy applications. In Energies (Vol. 9, Issue 8). MDPI AG. doi:10.3390/en9080607

Peters, J. F. (2017). *Foundations of computer vision: computational geometry, visual image structures and object shape detection* (Vol. 124). Springer. doi:10.1007/978-3-319-52483-2

PetersM. E.NeumannM.IyyerM.GardnerM.ClarkC.LeeK.ZettlemoyerL. (2018). *Deep contextualised word representations*. arXiv:1802.05365v2.

Peyser, T., Dassau, E., Breton, M., & Skyler, J. S. (2014). The artificial pancreas: Current status and future prospects in the management of diabetes. *Annals of the New York Academy of Sciences*, *1311*(1), 102–123. doi:10.1111/nyas.12431 PMID:24725149

Phan, D. H., Pointcheval, D., Shahandashti, S. F., & Strefler, M. (2013). Adaptive CCA broadcast encryption with constant-size secret keys and ciphertexts. *International Journal of Information Security*, *12*(4), 251–265. doi:10.100710207-013-0190-0

Pineau, J., Bellemare, M. G., Rush, A. J., Ghizaru, A., & Murphy, S. A. (2007). Constructing evidence-based treatment strategies using methods from computer science. *Drug and Alcohol Dependence*, *88*, S52–S60. doi:10.1016/j.drugalcdep.2007.01.005 PMID:17320311

Pineau, J., Guez, A., Vincent, R., Panuccio, G., & Avoli, M. (2009). Treating epilepsy via adaptive neurostimulation: A reinforcement learning approach. *International Journal of Neural Systems*, *19*(04), 227–240. doi:10.1142/S0129065709001987 PMID:19731397

Piret, J., & Boivin, G. (2020). Pandemics throughout history. *Frontiers in Microbiology*, *11*, 631736. doi:10.3389/fmicb.2020.631736 PMID:33584597

Pournader, M., Shi, Y., Seuring, S., & Koh, S. L. (2020). Blockchain applications in supply chains, transport and logistics: A systematic review of the literature. *International Journal of Production Research*, *58*(7), 2063–2081. doi:10.1080/00207543.2019.1650976

Prakash, R. (2019). Cyber crime: A critical study. *International Journal of Legal Developments and Allied Issues, 5*(5), 163-171. https://thelawbrigade.com/wp-content/uploads/2019/09/Rohit-prakash.pdf

Prasad, G., Jain, A. K., Jain, P., & Nagesh, H. R. (2019). A Novel Approach to Optimize the Performance of Hadoop Frameworks for Sentiment Analysis. *International Journal of Open Source Software and Processes*, *10*(4), 44–59. doi:10.4018/IJOSSP.2019100103

Praveen Gujjar, J., & Prasanna Kumar, H. R. (2021). Image classification and prediction using transfer learning in colab notebook. *Global Transitions Proceedings, 2*(2), 382-385. doi:10.1016/j.gltp.2021.08.068

Praveen Gujjar, J., Prasanna Kumar, H. R., & Guru Prasad, M. S. (2023). Advanced NLP Framework for Text Processing. *6th International Conference on Information Systems and Computer Networks (ISCON)*, 1-3. 10.1109/ISCON57294.2023.10112058

Principle component analysis. (n.d.). https://www.javatpoint.com/principal-component-analysis

Compilation of References

Ptaszynski, M., Masui, F., Nakajima, Y., Kimura, Y., Rzepka, R., & Araki, K. (2016). *Detecting cyberbullying with morphosemantic patterns.* Paper presented at joint 8th international conference on soft computing and intelligent systems and 17th international symposium on advanced intelligent systems, Sapporo, Japan.

Radoglou-Grammatikis, P., Sarigiannidis, P., Efstathopoulos, G., Lagkas, T., Fragulis, G., & Sarigiannidis, A. (2021, June 1). A Self-Learning Approach for Detecting Intrusions in Healthcare Systems. *IEEE International Conference on Communications.* 10.1109/ICC42927.2021.9500354

Raisi, E., & Huang, B. (2016). *Cyberbullying identification using participant-vocabulary consistency.* Paper presented at 2016 ICML workshop on #Data4Good: Machine learning in social good applications, New York, NY.

Ramesh, R., & Revathy, N. (2017). Public auditing for shared data with efficient user revocation in the cloud. *International Journal for Advance Research and Development, 2*(5), 184–189.

Random forest algorithm. (n.d.). https://www.javatpoint.com/machine-learning-random-forest-algorithm

Rawat, K., Kumari, P., & Saha, L. (2021). COVID-19 vaccine: A recent update in pipeline vaccines, their design and development strategies. *European Journal of Pharmacology, 892,* 173751. doi:10.1016/j.ejphar.2020.173751 PMID:33245898

Rawat, V., Gulati, K., Kaur, U., Seth, J. K., Solanki, V., Venkatesh, A. N., Singh, D. P., Singh, N., & Loganathan, M. (2022). A Supervised Learning Identification System for Prognosis of Breast Cancer. *Mathematical Problems in Engineering, 2022,* 1–8. doi:10.1155/2022/7459455

Razdan, S., & Sharma, S. (2021). Internet of Medical Things (IoMT): Overview, Emerging Technologies, and Case Studies. In IETE Technical Review (Institution of Electronics and Telecommunication Engineers, India). Taylor and Francis Ltd. doi:10.1080/02564602.2021.1927863

Reddy, B. V., Krishna, G. J., Ravi, V., & Dasgupta, D. (2021). *Machine learning and feature selection based ransomware detection using hexacodes. In evolution in computational intelligence.* Springer.

Regression analysis in machine learning. (n.d.). https://www.javatpoint.com/regression-analysis-in-machine-learning

Rid, T. (2012). Cyber war will not take place. *The Journal of Strategic Studies, 35*(1), 5–32. doi:10.1080/01402390.2011.608939

Rizwan, K. (2021). HarX: Real-time harassment detection tool using machine learning. In *2021 International Conference of Modern Trends in Information and Communication Technology Industry (MTICTI).* IEEE. 10.1109/MTICTI53925.2021.9664755

Rui, W., Xing, K., & Jia, Y. (2016). BOWL: Bag of word clusters text representation using word embeddings. In *Proc. International Conference on Knowledge Science, Engineering and Management.* 10.1007/978-3-319-47650-6_1

Ruj, S., Stojmenovic, M., & Nayak, A. (2013). Decentralized access control with anonymous authentication of data stored in clouds. *IEEE Transactions on Parallel and Distributed Systems*, *25*(2), 384–394. doi:10.1109/TPDS.2013.38

Runciman, B. (2020). Cybersecurity report 2020. *Itnow*, *62*(4), 28–29. doi:10.1093/itnow/bwaa103

Rush, A. J., Fava, M., Wisniewski, S. R., Lavori, P. W., Trivedi, M. H., Sackeim, H. A., Thase, M. E., Nierenberg, A. A., Quitkin, F. M., Kashner, T. M., Kupfer, D. J., Rosenbaum, J. F., Alpert, J., Stewart, J. W., McGrath, P. J., Biggs, M. M., Shores-Wilson, K., Lebowitz, B. D., Ritz, L., & Niederehe, G.the STAR*D Investigators Group. (2004). Sequenced treatment alternatives to relieve depression (star* d): Rationale and design. *Controlled Clinical Trials*, *25*(1), 119–142. doi:10.1016/S0197-2456(03)00112-0 PMID:15061154

Sabukunze, I. D., Setyohadi, D. B., & Sulistyoningsih, M. (2021, April). Designing an IoT based smart monitoring and emergency alert system for COVID19 patients. In *2021 6th International Conference for Convergence in Technology (I2CT)* (pp. 1-5). IEEE. 10.1109/I2CT51068.2021.9418078

Sadiq, S., Mehmood, A., Ullah, S., Ahmad, M., Choi, G. S., & On, B.-W. (2021). Aggression detection through deep neural model on Twitter. *Future Generation Computer Systems*, *114*, 120–129. doi:10.1016/j.future.2020.07.050

Sanger, D. E., & Mazzetti, M. (2016). US had cyberattack plan if Iran nuclear dispute led to conflict. *New York Times, 16.*

Sarker, I. H., Kayes, A. S. M., Badsha, S., Alqahtani, H., Watters, P., & Ng, A. (2020). Cybersecurity data science: An overview from machine learning perspective. *Journal of Big Data*, *7*(1), 41. Advance online publication. doi:10.118640537-020-00318-5

Schaefer, A. J., Bailey, M. D., Shechter, S. M., & Roberts, M. S. (2005). *Modeling medical treatment using markov decision processes. In Operations Research and Health Care.* Springer.

Schmitz, P., Hildebrandt, J., Valdez, A. C., Kobbelt, L., & Ziefle, M. (2018). You spin my head right round: Threshold of limited immersion for rotation gains in redirected walking. *IEEE Transactions on Visualization and Computer Graphics*, *24*(4), 1623–1632. doi:10.1109/TVCG.2018.2793671 PMID:29543179

Sengan, S., Khalaf, O. I., Vidya Sagar, P., Sharma, D. K., Arokia Jesu Prabhu, L., & Hamad, A. A. (2022). Secured and Privacy-Based IDS for Healthcare Systems on E-Medical Data Using Machine Learning Approach. *International Journal of Reliable and Quality E-Healthcare*, *11*(3), 1–11. doi:10.4018/IJRQEH.289175

Seo, J. H., & Emura, K. (2013). Revocable identity-based encryption revisited: Security model and construction. *Public-Key Cryptography–PKC 2013: 16th International Conference on Practice and Theory in Public-Key Cryptography, Nara, Japan, February 26–March 1, 2013 Proceedings*, *16*, 216–234.

Sharma, M. K. (2011). *Cyber Warfare: The Power of the Unseen.* KW Publ.

Shone, N., Ngoc, T. N., Phai, V. D., & Shi, Q. (n.d.). *A Deep Learning Approach to Network Intrusion Detection.* Retrieved September 2, 2022, from https://ieeexplore.ieee.org/document/8264962

Si-Ahmed A. Al-Garadi M. A. Boustia N. (2022). Survey of Machine Learning Based Intrusion Detection Methods for Internet of Medical Things. *ArXiv Preprint.* https://arxiv.org/abs/2202.09657

Singer, P. W., & Friedman, A. (2014). *Cybersecurity: What everyone needs to know.* OUP USA.

Singh, P., Tripathi, V., Singh, K. D., Guru Prasad, M. S., & Aditya Pai, H. (2023, April). A Task Scheduling Algorithm for Optimizing Quality of Service in Smart Healthcare System. In *International Conference on IoT, Intelligent Computing and Security: Select Proceedings of IICS 2021* (pp. 43-50). Singapore: Springer Nature Singapore. 10.1007/978-981-19-8136-4_4

Singhal, P., & Bansal, A. (2013). Improved textual cyberbullying detection using data mining. *International Journal of Information and Computation Technology, 3*(6), 569–575.

Singh, N., Singh, D. P., & Pant, B. (2017). A Comprehensive Study of Big Data Machine Learning Approaches and Challenges. *2017 International Conference on Next Generation Computing and Information Systems (ICNGCIS)*, 80–85. 10.1109/ICNGCIS.2017.14

Sittig, D. F., & Singh, H. (2016). A socio-technical approach to preventing, mitigating, and recovering from ransomware attacks. *Applied Clinical Informatics, 7*(02), 624–632. doi:10.4338/ACI-2016-04-SOA-0064 PMID:27437066

Soliman, Y. M. (2014). *Personalized medical treatments using novel reinforcement learning algorithms.* arXiv preprint arXiv:1406.3922

Soundar, K. R., & Ponesakki, P. (2016). Cyberbullying Detection based on text representation. *International Journal of Engineering Science, 6*(10), 2776–2785.

Srinivasakumar, V., Vanamoorthy, M., Sairaj, S., & Ganesh, S. (2022). An alternative C++-based HPC system for Hadoop MapReduce. *Open Computer Science, 12*(1), 238–247. doi:10.1515/comp-2022-0246

Statistical Language – Correlation and Causation at Australian Bureau of Statistics. (n.d.). https://www.abs.gov.au/

Steed, D. (2015). The Strategic Implications of Cyber Warfare. In A. Green James (Ed.), *Cyber Warfare A multidisciplinary analysis.* Library of Congress Cataloging-in-Publication Data. doi:10.4324/9781315761565-5

Stevens, F., Nurse, J. R., & Arief, B. (2021). Cyber stalking, cyber harassment and adult mental health: A systematic review. *Cyberpsychology, Behavior, and Social Networking, 24*(6), 367–376. doi:10.1089/cyber.2020.0253 PMID:33181026

Stieg, C. (2020). *How this Canadian start-up spotted coronavirus before everyone else knew about it.* CNBC.

Stiennon, R. (2015). *There Will Be Cyberwar: b How the Move to Network-Centric Warfighting Set The Stage For Cyberwar*. IT-Harvest Press.

Strielkina, A., Illiashenko, O., Zhydenko, M., & Uzun, D. (2018). Cybersecurity of healthcare IoT-based systems: regulation and case-oriented assessment. *2018 IEEE 9th International Conference on Dependable Systems, Services and Technologies (DESSERT)*, 67–73. 10.1109/DESSERT.2018.8409101

Subasi, A., Algebsani, S., Alghamdi, W., Kremic, E., Almaasrani, J., & Abdulaziz, N. (2021). Intrusion Detection in Smart Healthcare Using Bagging Ensemble Classifier. In CMBEBIH 2021 (pp. 164–171). doi:10.1007/978-3-030-73909-6_18

Sun, G., Matsui, T., Hakozaki, Y., & Abe, S. (2015). An infectious disease/fever screening radar system which stratifies higher-risk patients within ten seconds using a neural network and the fuzzy grouping method. *The Journal of Infection*, *70*(3), 230–236. doi:10.1016/j.jinf.2014.12.007 PMID:25541528

Support vector machine algorithm. (n.d.). https://www.javatpoint.com/machine-learning-support-vector-machine-algorithm

Tavallaee, M., Bagheri, E., Lu, W., & Ghorbani, A. A. (n.d.). *A detailed analysis of the KDD CUP 99 data set*. Retrieved September 1, 2022, from https://ieeexplore.ieee.org/document/5356528

Tesfahun, A., & Bhaskari, D. L. (n.d.). *Intrusion Detection Using Random Forests Classifier with SMOTE and Feature Reduction*. Retrieved September 1, 2022, from https://ieeexplore.ieee.org/document/6701490

Tgavalekos, K., Namayanja, J. M., & Alhassan, R. (2018). Characterization of network behavior to detect changes. *Proceedings of the Workshop Program of the 19th International Conference on Distributed Computing and Networking*, 1–6. 10.1145/3170521.3170523

Thamer, N., & Alubady, R. (2021, April). A Survey of Ransomware Attacks for Healthcare Systems: Risks, Challenges, Solutions and Opportunity of Research. In *2021 1st Babylon International Conference on Information Technology and Science (BICITS)* (pp. 210-216). IEEE.

Thamer, N., & Alubady, R. (2021). A Survey of Ransomware Attacks for Healthcare Systems: Risks, Challenges, Solutions and Opportunity of Research. *1st Babylon International Conference on Information Technology and Science (BICITS)*, 210-216. 10.1109/BICITS51482.2021.9509877

Thamer, N., & Alubady, R. (2021). A Survey of Ransomware Attacks for Healthcare Systems: Risks, Challenges, Solutions and Opportunity of Research. *International Journal on Computer Science and Engineering*, *6*(1), 80–85.

Thamilarasu, G., Odesile, A., & Hoang, A. (2020). An Intrusion Detection System for Internet of Medical Things. *IEEE Access : Practical Innovations, Open Solutions*, *8*, 181560–181576. doi:10.1109/ACCESS.2020.3026260

Thanh Nguyen, P., Dang Bich Huynh, V., Dang Vo, K., Thanh Phan, P., Elhoseny, M., & Le, D.-N. (2021). Deep Learning based Optimal Multimodal Fusion Framework for Intrusion Detection Systems for Healthcare Data. *Computers, Materials & Continua, 66*(3), 2555–2571. doi:10.32604/cmc.2021.012941

The Computer Algorithm That Was Among the First to Detect the Coronavirus Outbreak. (n.d.). http://www.cnbnews.com

The National Crime Records Bureau. Crime in India. (2020). https://www.thehinducentre.com /resources/ article36608197.ece/binary/CII%202020%20 Volume%201.pdf

The Statista. (2021a). *Number of internet users in India.* Available at: https://www.statista.com/ statistics/255146/number-of-internet-users-in-india/

The Statista. (2021b). *Number of social network users in India.* Available at: https://www.statista. com/statistics/278407/number-of-social-network-users-in-india

The, U. S. (2022, May 19). *Government and the World Health Organization.* https://www.kff. org/coronavirus-covid-19/fact-sheet/the-u-s-government-and-the-world-health-organization/

Thomas, L., & Bhat, S. (2021). Machine Learning and Deep Learning Techniques for IoT-based Intrusion Detection Systems: A Literature Review. *International Journal of Management, Technology, and Social Sciences, 6*(2), 296–314. doi:10.5281/zenodo.5814702

Time of India website: Two arrested for cyberstalking. (2021). Available at: https://timesofindia. indiatimes.com/city/hyderabad/two-arrested-for-cyber-stalking/ articleshow/ 82280780.cms

Times of India. (2021). *Beware! Cyberstalking is on the rise during the pandemic.* Available at: https://timesofindia.indiatimes.com/life-style/spotlight/beware-cyberstalking-is-on-the-rise-during-the-pandemic/articleshow/81924158.cms

Toghuj, W., & Turab, N. (2022). A survey on security threats in the internet of medical things (IoMT). *Journal of Theoretical and Applied Information Technology, 100*(10). www.jatit.org

Tolba, M., Ouadfel, S., & Meshoul, S. (2021). Hybrid ensemble approaches to online harassment detection in highly imbalanced data. *Expert Systems with Applications, 175,* 114751. doi:10.1016/j. eswa.2021.114751

Tomar, P., Kaur, G., & Singh, P. (2018). A prototype of IoT-based real time smart street parking system for smart cities. In *Internet of things and big data analytics toward next-generation intelligence* (pp. 243–263). Springer. doi:10.1007/978-3-319-60435-0_10

Tosh, D. K., Shetty, S., Liang, X., Kamhoua, C. A., Kwiat, K. A., & Njilla, L. (2017, May). Security implications of blockchain cloud with analysis of block withholding attack. In *2017 17th IEEE/ACM International Symposium on Cluster, Cloud and Grid Computing (CCGRID)* (pp. 458-467). IEEE. 10.1109/CCGRID.2017.111

Truman, J. L. (2010). *Examining intimate partner stalking and use of technology in stalking victimisation* [Ph.D. thesis]. University of Central Florida Orlando, FL.

Tsai, C. W., Lai, C. F., Chiang, M. C., & Yang, L. T. (2013). Data mining for internet of things: a survey. *IEEE Communications Surveys & Tutorials, 16*(1), 77-97.

Tschoellitsch, T., Dünser, M., Böck, C., Schwarzbauer, K., & Meier, J. (2021, March). Machine learning prediction of SARS-CoV-2 polymerase chain reaction results with routine blood tests. *Laboratoriums Medizin 15, 52*(2), 146–149. doi:10.1093/labmed/lmaa111

Tully, J., Selzer, J., Phillips, J. P., O'Connor, P., & Dameff, C. (2020). Healthcare challenges in the era of cybersecurity. *Health Security, 18*(3), 228–231. doi:10.1089/hs.2019.0123 PMID:32559153

Understanding random forest. (n.d.). https://www.analyticsvidhya.com/blog/2021/06/understanding-random-forest/

Usak, M., Kubiatko, M., Shabbir, M. S., Viktorovna Dudnik, O., Jermsittiparsert, K., & Rajabion, L. (2020). Health care service delivery based on the Internet of things: A systematic and comprehensive study. *International Journal of Communication Systems, 33*(2), e4179. doi:10.1002/dac.4179

Vaiyapuri, T., Binbusayyis, A., & Varadarajan, V. (2021). Security, Privacy and Trust in IoMT Enabled Smart Healthcare System: A Systematic Review of Current and Future Trends. *IJACSA). International Journal of Advanced Computer Science and Applications, 12*(2), 731–737. doi:10.14569/IJACSA.2021.0120291

Vanamoorthy, M., & Chinnaiah, V. (2020). Congestion-free transient plane (CFTP) using bandwidth sharing during link failures in SDN. *The Computer Journal, 63*(6), 832–843. doi:10.1093/comjnl/bxz137

Venter, I. M., Blignaut, R. J., Renaud, K., & Venter, M. A. (2019). Cyber security education is as essential as "the three R's". *Heliyon, 5*(12), e02855. doi:10.1016/j.heliyon.2019.e02855 PMID:31872107

Vijayarani, & Ilamathi, & Nithya. (2015). Pre-processing techniques for text mining-an overview. *International Journal of Computer Science & Communication Networks, 5*(1), 7–16.

Villora, B., Yubero, S., & Navarro, R. (2020). Subjective well-being among victimised university students: Comparison between cyber dating abuse and bullying victimisation. *Information Technology & People*. Advance online publication. doi:10.1108/ITP-11-2018-0535

Vincent, P., Larochelle, H., Larochelle, H., Bengio, Y., & Manzagol, P. (2010, March 1). Stacked Denoising Autoencoders: Learning Useful Representations in a Deep Network with a Local Denoising Criterion. *The Journal of Machine Learning Research*. https://dl.acm.org/doi/10.5555/1756006.1953039

Wang, C., Chow, S. S., Wang, Q., Ren, K., & Lou, W. (2011). Privacy-preserving public auditing for secure cloud storage. *IEEE Transactions on Computers, 62*(2), 362–375. doi:10.1109/TC.2011.245

Wang, S., Ouyang, L., Yuan, Y., Ni, X., Han, X., & Wang, F. Y. (2019). Blockchain-enabled smart contracts: Architecture, applications, and future trends. *IEEE Transactions on Systems, Man, and Cybernetics. Systems, 49*(11), 2266–2277. doi:10.1109/TSMC.2019.2895123

Compilation of References

Wani, A., & Revathi, S. (2020). Ransomware protection in IoT using software defined networking. *Iranian Journal of Electrical and Computer Engineering, 10*(3), 3166–3175.

Wing, Ng, Zeng, & Zhang. (2016, June 21). *Dual autoencoder features for imbalance classification problem.* https://www.sciencedirect.com/science/article/abs/pii/S0031320316301303

Wolfers, A. (1952). "National security" as an ambiguous symbol. *Political Science Quarterly, 67*(4), 481–502. doi:10.2307/2145138

World Health Organization. (n.d.). *Coronavirus (COVID-19) dashboard.* https://covid19.who.int/table

Wüst, K., & Gervais, A. (2018, June). Do you need a blockchain? In *2018 Crypto Valley Conference on Blockchain Technology (CVCBT)* (pp. 45-54). IEEE. 10.1109/CVCBT.2018.00011

Xu, S. (2018). Bayesian Naïve Bayes classifiers to text classification. *Journal of Information Science, 44*(1), 48–59. doi:10.1177/0165551516677946

Yadav, S., Gulia, P., Gill, N. S., & Chatterjee, J. M. (2022). A real-time crowd monitoring and management system for social distance classification and healthcare using deep learning. *Journal of Healthcare Engineering.* . doi:10.1155/2022/2130172

Yamany, B. (2022). *A New Scheme for Ransomware Classification and Clustering Using Static Features.* MDPI. www.mdpi.com/2079-9292/11/20/3307/html

Yang, K., & Jia, X. (2012). An efficient and secure dynamic auditing protocol for data storage in cloud computing. *IEEE Transactions on Parallel and Distributed Systems, 24*(9), 1717–1726. doi:10.1109/TPDS.2012.278

Yasini, S., Naghibi Sistani, M. B., & Karimpour, A. (2009). Agent-based simulation for blood glucose. *International Journal of Applied Science, Engineering and Technology, 5,* 89–95.

Yates, J. A. (2013). *Cyber Warfare: An Evolution in Warfare not Just War Theory.* Marine Corps Command.

Zainudin, N. M., Zainal, K. H., Hasbullah, N. A., Wahab, N. A., & Ramli, S. (2016). A review on cyberbullying in Malaysia from a digital forensic perspective. *Proc. International Conference on Information and Communication Technology,* 246-250. 10.1109/ICICTM.2016.7890808

Zakus, D., Bhattacharyya, O., & Wei, X. (2014). Health systems, management, and organization in global health. In *Understanding Global Health* (2nd ed.). McGrawHill. https://accessmedicine.mhmedical.com/content.aspx?bookid=710&sectionid=46796921

Zarpelao, B. B., Miani, R. S., Kawakami, C. T., & de Alvarenga, S. C. (2017, February 21). *A survey of intrusion detection in Internet of Things.* https://www.sciencedirect.com/science/article/abs/pii/S1084804517300802#!

Zee News website: Bulli Bai Controversy. (2021). https://zeenews.india.com/india/bulli-bai-controversy-all-you-need-to-know-about-the-app-targeting-muslim-women-on-social-media-2424831.html

Zhang, Q., Yang, L., Chen, Z., & Li, P. (2018, January 1). *A survey on deep learning for big data.* https://www.semanticscholar.org/paper/A-survey-on-deep-learning-for-big-data-Zhang-Yang/b7919fadb4c1bf959b1e410463594afacfda7dc6

Zhao, Y., Kosorok, M. R., & Zeng, D. (2009). Reinforcement learning design for cancer clinical trials. *Statistics in Medicine*, *28*(26), 3294–3315. doi:10.1002im.3720 PMID:19750510

Zhong, F., Xing, J., Li, X., Liu, X., Fu, Z., Xiong, Z., Lu, D., Wu, X., Zhao, J., Tan, X., Li, F., Luo, X., Li, Z., Chen, K., Zheng, M., & Jiang, H. (2018). Artificial intelligence in drug design. *Science China. Life Sciences*, *61*(10), 1191–1204. doi:10.100711427-018-9342-2 PMID:30054833

Zhong, H., Li, H., Squicciarini, A. C., Rajtmajer, S. M., Griffin, C., Miller, D. J., & Caragea, C. (2016, July). Content-Driven Detection of Cyberbullying on the Instagram Social Network. *IJCAI (United States)*, *16*, 3952–3958.

Zhu, S., Cai, Z., Hu, H., Li, Y., & Li, W. (2019). zkCrowd: A hybrid blockchain-based crowdsourcing platform. *IEEE Transactions on Industrial Informatics*, *16*(6), 4196–4205. doi:10.1109/TII.2019.2941735

Zou, Y., Meng, T., Zhang, P., Zhang, W., & Li, H. (2020). Focus on blockchain: A comprehensive survey on academic and application. *IEEE Access : Practical Innovations, Open Solutions*, *8*, 187182–187201. doi:10.1109/ACCESS.2020.3030491

About the Contributors

Abhishek Bansal received the MCA degree from Dr. B. R. Ambedkar University, Agra, Uttar Pradesh, India, in 2004 and Ph.D. degree from University of Delhi, Delhi in 2017. he joined Paliwal (PG) college, Shikohabad as lecturer in 2007. He was awarded with UGC NET-JRF in June 2009/December 2009. In 2012, He has joined as Assistant Professor in Department of Computer Science, Indira Gandhi National Tribal University, Amarkantak, Madhya Pradesh, India and currently working as Senior Assistant Professor. He has more than 14 years of teaching and research experience. His research interest is in information security, cyber security and machine learning. He has published more than 20 research papers in reputed journals like IEEE, springer, Taylor & Frances, IGI Global and many more.

Kritika Dhawale completed her B.Tech from IIIT Nagpur. She worked as a Deep Learning Engineer at Skylark Drones, Banglore. She presented research papers at IEEE conferences and published book chapters in IGI Global Publication. Currently, she is pursuing Master's in Data Science at the University of Technology Sydney.

Arvind Kumar Gautam was born in Rewa,Madhya Pradesh, India. He received his Master of Philosophy degree in Computer Science in 2009 from APS University, Rewa,Madhya Pradesh, India. He is a Ph.D. research scholar in the Department of Computer Science, Indira Gandhi National Tribal University, Amarkantak, Madhya Pradesh,India. He is also working as a System Analyst for 9 years at Indira Gandhi National Tribal University, Amarkantak, Madhya Pradesh. He has more than 10 years of working experience in server administration, networking, cybersecurity, web programming, and teaching. He has published several research papers in international journals and conferences. His academic research interests mainly include Cyber Security, Machine Learning,and Web Engineering.

Praveen Gujjar is an academician with 13 years of teaching experience. He has served in engineering and management institute. His research article is published in science direct.

Abhishek Kumar have been completed B.Tech in computer science engineering from motihari college of engineering east champaran and recently complted M.Tech in computer science & technology from school of computer & systems sciences jawaharlal nehru university new delhi. He has attend many workshop, conference, and also work as organising member of online ATAL faculty development program. my research area are Blockchain, cyber secuirty, network secuirty, and IoT. currently he has working as assistant software engineer in centre for railway information system under ministry of railways, Government of india.

Sudesh Kumar is currently working as an Assistant Professor in the Department of Computer Science at Indira Gandhi National Tribal University (A Central University), Amarkantak, Madhya Pradesh, India. He received his M.Sc. (Mathematics) and M.E. (Computer Science and Engineering) in 2005 and 2009, respectively. He obtained his PhD in Computer Science from the Faculty of Computer Science, Indira Gandhi National Tribal University, Madhya Pradesh, India, in 2021. He worked as an Assistant Professor in the Department of Computer Science and Engineering, Central University of Rajasthan, India, from July 2010 to September 2012. He has more than 13 years of teaching, administrative and research experience. Currently, he is associated with a wide range of journals and conferences as chief editor, editor, chair and member. His current research interest includes Flying Ad-hoc Networks, Vehicular Ad hoc Networks and Information Security. He is supervising many M. Tech., MCA and PhD students. Dr Kumar has published more than 20 research articles with good impact factors in reputed International Journals and Conferences, including IEEE, Elsevier, Springer, ICIC Express Letters, IGI Global etc. Dr Kumar also is a member of various Professional Bodies and delivered many expert talks in reputed Universities and Institutes.

Devendra Rautela is pursuing Doctorate from Graphic Era Deemed to be University. His areas of interest are Deep Learning, Machine Learning, Soft computing and data mining. He has more than 10 publications in reputed National and International SCOPUS, UGC Approve Journals and conferences. Currently he is working as Assistant professor in Graphic Era Hill University Bhimtal. He has an experience of around 06 years of teaching.

Muthumanikandan V., B.E., M.E., Ph.D., is working as a Senior Assistant Professor(Grade II) in the School of Computing Science and Engineering, at Vellore Institute of Technology, Chennai, India. He received his B.E and M.E degree in Computer Science and Engineering discipline. He received his Ph.D degree in Computer Science and Engineering from MIT Campus, Anna University. His areas of interests include Networking, Software Defined Networking and Network Function Virtualization. He published many papers i reputed journals and conferences.

Index

A

Accuracy 15, 18-20, 23-25, 44, 65-66, 86, 90, 92-93, 125-126, 129-132, 135, 157, 159, 165
AES algorithm 72
Auditing 49, 74, 83-84
Authentication 3, 11, 18-20, 31, 46, 57, 65, 73, 75, 78, 84
Automatic Detection 140, 143, 155, 157-158, 165

B

Blockchain 10-11, 13, 20, 30-44, 46-51, 63-64, 66-67, 69

C

Classification models 15, 17
Computational Algorithms 131-132
Coping Strategies 143, 165-166
Critical Care 105, 117
Cyber Security 1, 8, 16-17, 51, 56-57, 70, 96, 98-102
Cyber Security Attack 51
Cyber-Attacks 2-3, 5-6, 8-9, 11, 17, 19, 23, 25-26, 67
Cyberbullying 143-144, 148-151, 157-158, 166-171
Cyberspace 96-100, 102-103
Cyberstalking 143-146, 148-170

D

Data Analytics 1, 7, 64, 105-106, 134, 139, 142
Disease Control 121
Disease Spread 128

E

E-Healthcare 28, 85-86
Encryption 2-3, 5-6, 9, 55, 72-73, 76-77, 79-84

H

Healthcare 1-14, 16-21, 24-31, 39, 42, 44-49, 51-58, 60-67, 69-70, 85-87, 94, 106, 108-109, 114-116, 124, 132, 134, 140, 142
Healthcare System 14, 16-19, 21, 25, 29-31, 39, 42, 44-47, 51, 56, 94

I

IDS 20-21, 25, 28, 85-89, 154
Information Security 48, 51, 63, 83, 168
Information Sharing 30-31, 47-48, 57
IoMT 15-20, 25, 27-29
IoT 5, 14, 16, 18-19, 25, 27, 30-31, 40, 42-44, 47-50, 63, 67, 69, 87-89, 93-94, 139

K

Key Management 31, 45-47, 79, 82
KNN 18-19, 23, 85, 89-90, 93, 122, 138

M

Machine Learning 2, 5, 10, 12, 15-18, 20-21,
23, 25-29, 51, 63, 65, 67-69, 85, 87-88,
90-91, 93-95, 105-106, 108, 115-118,
120, 122, 124, 126, 128-130, 132-134,
136-139, 141-143, 155-164, 166-169
Machine Learning Techniques 67, 85, 87,
105, 120, 157-158, 167
Mental Disorder 105, 115

N

National Security 96-100, 102-104

P

Pandemic 30-31, 47, 120-121, 127, 129-
130, 132-135, 150, 170
Payment Gateway 72
Phishing Attack 57-59

Privacy 2, 5-6, 8-11, 18, 20, 25-27, 29,
35, 48, 50, 56, 67, 73-76, 79-80, 82-
83, 160

R

Ransomware Attacks 3, 51-52, 63-64, 66,
68, 70
Regression models 15, 17, 23, 25, 27
Reinforcement Learning 105-109, 115-119

S

Security Key 72
Storage 16, 19, 31, 37-38, 40, 60, 68, 73-74,
76, 79, 81-84, 88

V

Victims 59-61, 143, 145-146, 150, 152-155,
160, 164-166
Visualization 18, 70

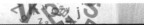
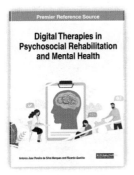
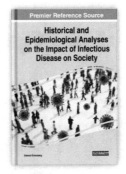
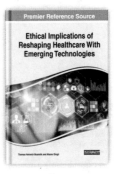
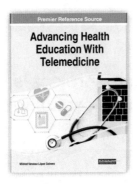
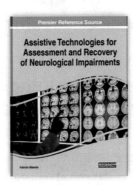
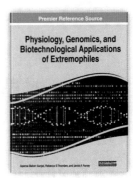
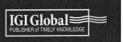

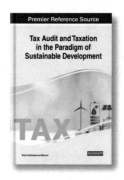
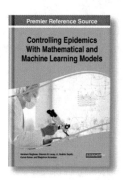
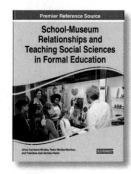
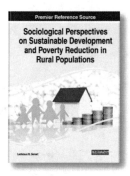

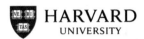 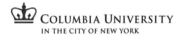 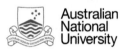
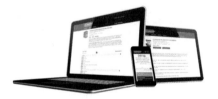

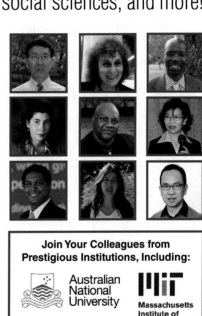

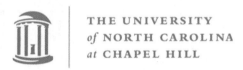
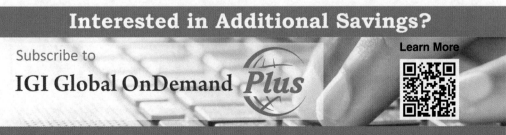

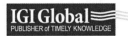
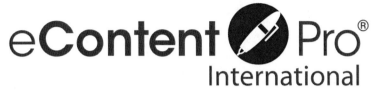
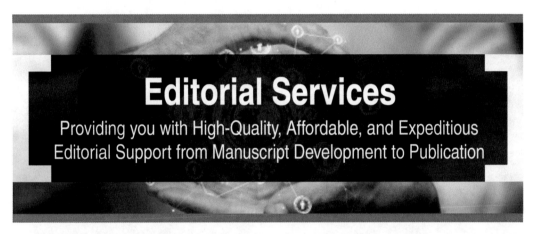

Printed in the United States
by Baker & Taylor Publisher Services